£5.99.

OXFORD CARDIOLOGY LIBRARY

Acute Coronary Syndromes

Acute Coronary Syndromes

Edited by

Dr Graham Jackson

FRCP, FESC, FACC,
Consultant Cardiologist,
Guy's and St Thomas NHS Foundation Trust,
London, UK

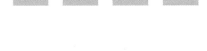

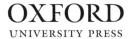

OXFORD

UNIVERSITY PRESS

OXFORD
UNIVERSITY PRESS

Great Clarendon Street, Oxford OX2 6DP

Oxford University Press is a department of the University of Oxford.
It furthers the University's objective of excellence in research, scholarship,
and education by publishing worldwide in

Oxford New York

Auckland Cape Town Dar es Salaam Hong Kong Karachi
Kuala Lumpur Madrid Melbourne Mexico City Nairobi
New Delhi Shanghai Taipei Toronto

With offices in

Argentina Austria Brazil Chile Czech Republic France Greece
Guatemala Hungary Italy Japan Poland Portugal Singapore
South Korea Switzerland Thailand Turkey Ukraine Vietnam

Oxford is a registered trade mark of Oxford University Press
in the UK and in certain other countries

Published in the United States
by Oxford University Press Inc., New York

British Library Cataloguing in Publication Data

Data available

Library of Congress Cataloging in Publication Data

Data available

Typeset by Newgen Imaging Systems (P) Ltd., Chennai, India
Printed in Italy
on acid-free paper by
Legoprint S.p.A

ISBN 978-0-19-954349-6

10 9 8 7 6 5 4 3 2 1

616.12
JAC

Contents

Contributors

Professor Martin R Bennett
MA, PhD, FRCP, FmedSci,
BHF Professor of Cardiovascular
Sciences and Honorary
Consultant Cardiologist,
Division of Cardiovascular
Medicine, Addenbrooke's
Centre for Clinical Investigation,
Addenbrooke's Hospital,
Cambridge, UK

Dr Nick Boon
Consultant Cardiologist,
Royal Infirmary of Edinburgh,
Edinburgh, UK

Patrick Calvert

Dr Shui Hao Chin
MA, MRCP,
Cardiology Specialist Registrar

Dr Brian Clapp
Consultant Cardiologist,
Guy's and St Thomas' NHS
Foundation Trust, London, UK

Dr Derek Leslie Connolly
PhD, FRCP,
Consultant Cardiologist and
Honorary Senior Clinical Lecturer,
Sandwell & West Birmingham
Hospitals NHS Trust and the
University of Birmingham,
Birmingham, UK

Dr Peter Henriksen
Consultant Cardiologist,
Western General Hospital,
Edinburgh, UK

Dr Kevin Jennings
FRCP, Consultant Cardiologist,
Aberdeen Royal Infirmary,
Aberdeen, UK

Professor MG Kirby
Visiting Professor,
Faculty of Health & Human
Sciences, Centre for Research
in Primary and Community
Care (CRIPACC), University of
Hertfordshire, Hatfield,
London, UK

Dr Gregory YH Lip
FRCP, Professor of
Cardiovascular Medicine,
Department of Medicine,
City Hospital,
Birmingham, UK

Professor Michael Marber
Professor of Cardiology,
The Rayne Institute,
King's College,
University of London, UK

Dr Andrew A. McCleod
FRCP, FESC,
Consultant Cardiologist

Samir Srivastava
MRCP, Research Fellow

Dr Ian Webb
BHF Clinical Research Fellow,
The Rayne Institute,
King's College,
University of London, UK

Dr Anthony S. Wierzbicki
Consultant in Specialist
Laboratory Medicine,
St Thomas' Hospital,
London, UK

Symbols and abbreviations

ACC	American College of Cardiology
ACCORD	Action to Control Cardiovascular Risk in Diabetes trial
ACE	Angiotensin-converting enzyme
ACE-I	Angiotension-converting enzyme inhibitor
ACS	Acute coronary syndromes
ADP	adenosine diphosphate
AF	atrial fibrillation
AHA	American Heart Association
AIM-HIGH	Atherothrombosis Intervention in Metabolic Syndrome with Low HDL/High Triglycerides and Impact on Global Health Outcomes trial
ALLHAT	Antihypertensive Lipid-Lowering treatment to prevent Heart Attack Trial
ARB	angiotension receptor blocker
ASCOT	Anglo-Scandinavian Coronary Outcomes study
ASSIST	Assessment of Implementation Strategies
AV	atrioventricular
A-Z	Aggrastat to Zocor trial
BACR	British Association for Cardiac Rehabilitation
BHS	British Hypertension Society
BMA	British Medical Association
BMI	body mass index
CABG	coronary artery bypass grafting
CAD	coronary artery disease
CAPRIE	Clopidogrel versus Aspirin in Patients at Risk for Ischemic Events trial
CCB	Calcium channel blocker
CCU	Coronary Care Unit
CHARISMA	Clopidogrel for High Atherothrombotic Risk and Ischemic Stabilization, Management and Avoidance
CHD	coronary heart disease
CI	cardiac index

CKD	Chronic kidney disease
CK-MB	Creatine Kinase MB cardioselective isoenzyme
COX-1	cyclooxygenase-1
CPAP	continuous positive airway pressure
CURE	Clopidogrel in Unstable angina to prevent Recurrent ischemic Events trial
CV	cardiovascular events
CR	cardiac rehabilitation
CRESCENDO	Comprehensive Rimonabant Evaluation Study of Cardiovascular ENDpoints and Outcomes
DART	Diet And Reinforction Trial
DASH	Diet and Sodium in Hypertension study
DCCV	Direct current cardioversion
DIGAMI	Diabetes Mellitus Insulin-Glucose Infusion in Acute Myocardial Infarction trial
DM	diabetes mellitus
ECG	electrocardiogram
EF	ejection fraction
EP	electrophysiology
EPHESUS	Eplerenone Post-Acute Myocardial Infarction Heart Failure Efficacy and Survival Study
ESPRIT	European/Australasian Stroke Prevention in Reversible Ischemic Trial
EUROPA	European trial On Reduction Of cardiac events with Perindopril in stable coronary Artery disease
FRISC	Fragmin and fast revascularization during instability in coronary artery disease.
GI	gastrointestinal
GISSI-P	Grouppo Italiano per lo Studio della Sopravivenza nell 'Infarto miocardio Prevenzione trial
GMS	General Medical Services
GPC	General Practitioners Committee
GRACE	Global Registry of Acute Coronary Events
GTN	glyceryl trinitrate
GUARANTEE	Global Unstable Angina Registry and Treatment Evaluation study
HDL	high-density lipoprotein

HDL-C	high-density lipoprotein-cholesterol
HOPE	Heart Outcomes Prevention Evaluation
HPSCG	Heart Protection Study Collaborative Group
IABP	intra-aortic balloon pump
ICD	implantable cardiac defibrillator
IHD	ischaemic heart disease
ISIS	International Study of Infarct Survival
IV	intravenous
JELIS	Japan EPA Lipid Intervention Study
LAD	left anterior descending
LDL	low-density lipoprotein
LDL-C	low-density lipoprotein-cholesterol
LIFE	Losartan Intervention For Endpoint Reduction
LV	left ventricular
LVEF	left ventricular ejection fraction
LVF	left ventricular failure
MI	myocardial infarction
MILIS	Multicenter Investigation of Limitation of Infarct Size
MIRACL	Myocardial Ischemia Reduction with Aggressive Cholesterol Lowering trial
MR	mitral regurgitation
MRFIT	Multiple Risk Factor Intervention Trial
NICE	National Institute for Health and Clinical Excellence
NSAID	Non-steroidal anti-inflammatory drug
NSF	National Services Framework
NSTEMI	Non-ST elevated myocardial infarction
NYHA	New York Heart Association
PAWP	pulmonary artery wedge pressure
PCI	percutaneous coronary interverntion
PCOs	Primary Care Organizations
PROactive	PROspective pioglitAzone Clinical Trial in macroVascular Events
PROVE-IT	Pravastatin or Atorvastatin Evaluation and Infection Therapy trial
PURSUIT	Platelet glycoprotein IIb/IIIa in Unstable angina: Receptor Suppression Using Integrilin Therapy

QMAS	Quality Management and Analysis System
RALES	Randomized Aldactone Evaluation Study
RECORD	Rosiglitazone Evaluated for Cardiac Outcomes and Regulation of Glycaemia in Diabetes trial
RF-IVUS	radiofrequency intravascular ultrasound
RR	relative risk
RV	right ventricular
SBP	systolic blood pressure
SCD	sudden cardiac death
SCOUT	Sibutramine Cardiovascular Outcomes Trial
SHOCK	SHould we emergently revascularize Occluded Coronaries for cardiogenic shocK study
SIGN	Scottish Intercollegiate Guidelines Network
STEMI	ST-elevated myocardial infarction
TCFA	thin-cap fibroatheromata
THRIVE	Treatment of HDL to Reduce the Incidence of Vascular Events trial
TIMI	Thrombolysis in myocardial infarction study group
VALIANT	Valsartan In Acute myocardial infarction trial
VALUE	Valsartan Antihypertensive Long-term Use Evaluation trial
VF	ventricular fibrillation
VSD	ventricular septal defect
VSMCs	vascular smooth muscle cells
VT	ventricular tachycardia
XENDOS	XENical in the prevention of Diabetes in Obese Subjects trial

Chapter 1

Acute coronary syndromes: the epidemiology

Kevin Jennings

> **Key points**
> - Coronary disease is common and threatening.
> - It is also common and threatening in women.
> - There are recognised reversible risk factors.
> - There are validated scoring tools to identify high risk.

1.1 Introduction: the size of the problem

Cardiovascular disease is the leading cause of death in the United Kingdom, being responsible for over 208,000 deaths annually; 101, 000 of these are due to acute coronary heart disease. Thus, about half of all deaths from cardiovascular disease are due to coronary heart disease. Coronary heart disease itself is the commonest cause of death in the UK, causing the death of 1 in 5 men and 1 in 6 women. It is also the commonest cause of premature death (death before the age of 75), in the UK: 20 per cent of premature deaths in men and 11 per cent of premature deaths in women result from this pathology; acute coronary disease caused 33,000 premature deaths in the UK in 2005 (British Heart Foundation 2007).

Acute coronary syndromes encompass a spectrum of unstable coronary artery diseases from unstable angina to transmural myocardial infarction (MI). All have a common aetiology in the formation of thrombus on an inflamed and complicated atheromatous plaque. The principles behind the presentation, investigation, and management of these syndromes are similar, with important distinctions depending on the category of acute coronary syndrome.

Health improvements throughout much of the world have increased life expectancy globally by an average of 20 years—from 46 years in 1950 to 66 years in 1998 (Sen & Bonita 2000). However, currently, about 80 per cent of the world's cardiovascular disease burden occurs in low-income and middle-income countries (Yusuf *et al.* 2004). Death rates from coronary disease have been falling in the UK since the 1970s: for those under the age of 75, these rates have fallen 24 per cent in the last 10 years. In those under 65 years of age, the fall has been 46 per cent. A study has shown that 58 per cent of this mortality reduction in the 1980s and 1990s was due to reduction in risk factors and particularly, smoking. Treatment was considered responsible for the remaining two-fifths of this mortality reduction (Unal *et al.* 2004). Whilst the death rate from coronary heart disease has been falling in the UK, it has fallen further in other countries: the death rate for men aged 35–74 fell by 42 per cent between 1990 and 2000 in the UK but by 48 per cent in Australia and by 54 per cent in Norway. However, in this period some countries in Eastern Europe (particularly, countries of the former USSR), have experienced an increased mortality from coronary disease: in Ukraine there has been an increase in coronary mortality for men and women of more than 60 per cent. In the UK, death rates are highest in Scotland and the North of England and lowest in the South of England. The premature death rate is 70 per cent higher for men in Scotland than in the South West of England and 80 per cent higher for women. The death rate has fallen faster for non-manual than for manual workers: at the end of the 1990s the mortality rate was 50 per cent higher for male manual workers than for males in non-manual occupations. At the same time the premature death rate for women was 73 per cent higher for manual workers than for women in non-manual employ-ment (British Heart Foundation 2007). There is an established and strong relationship between death from coronary disease and social deprivation: it is likely that this relates to an increased smoking habit and poor diet in this population. Additionally, some ethnic groups appear more vulnerable to coronary disease. South Asians living in the UK have an excess death rate from coronary disease. Information from the 1990s shows that the death rate for South Asians is 46 per cent higher for men and 51 per cent higher for women than the average rate. Some data suggest that risk factors may vary among these disparate populations: for example, data suggest that lipids may not be a major contributor to acute MI in South Asian Indians (Pais *et al.* 1996).

1.2 **Risk variables**

With advancing age the mortality rate from coronary disease increases sharply, such that there is a 15-fold increase from 35–44 years to 55–64 years in men and an approximately 30 times increase in mortality in women over these time periods. The likelihood is that the impact of aging is a result of accumulating risk factors over time.

Men aged 35–44 have a rate of coronary disease 5 or 6 times greater than women of this age group. This disparity lessens with increasing age, but women tend to have coronary disease about ten years later than men. Thus, women with coronary disease are likely to have more advanced or complex coronary disease because they tend to be older with more co-morbidity.

With increasing total cholesterol levels across the range, there is an increase in coronary risk. This atherogenic risk appears to act through low-density lipoprotein (LDL)-cholesterol becoming oxidised and deposited in the coronary circulation. On the other hand, low levels of high-density lipoprotein (HDL)-cholesterol are known to be associated with enhanced coronary risk so higher levels of this lipid subfraction are considered desirable as 'protection' from coronary risk. Serum triglycerides have a positive relationship to the risk of coronary disease but are also closely and positively related to cholesterol and negatively to HDL-cholesterol. When these relationships are considered, triglycerides may have no influence independently on coronary risk.

Elevated blood pressure is an important and independent risk variable for coronary disease. Framingham has demonstrated a two-fold increase in the risk of coronary disease in those with blood pressure greater than 160/95 mmHg compared with those who are normotensive. This finding was confirmed in the British Regional Heart Study.

These studies have also demonstrated that the rate of coronary disease is about three times greater in smokers compared with those who have never smoked.

There is now compelling evidence that central obesity, as reflected by the waist/hip ratio, is associated with an independent risk of coronary disease. It is likely that this effect is mediated through known factors that occur co-morbidly with obesity including hypertension, unfavourable lipid profiles, insulin resistance reduced, and lack of physical exercise. There is accumulating evidence that regular physical activity protects against coronary events. The falling rates for mortality from coronary disease have been accompanied by an increase in obesity, paradoxically, possibly at least connected to a reduction in smoking and increased availability of better diets. In populations with increasing obesity, where diets do not lead to raised average levels of LDL-cholesterol, the absolute risk of coronary death is not increased. The potential threat from resulting diabetes, however, warns of the possibility of a reversal of the decreasing mortality from coronary disease in the light of a clear relationship between diabetes and vascular disease. In countries where coronary disease is prevalent, diabetes is associated with a two-fold increase in the risk of coronary events.

A family history of premature coronary disease in a first-degree relative is acknowledged to be an independent risk factor for coronary disease.

Pre-existing coronary disease increases the risk of coronary events: there is a six-fold increase in the risk of a myocardial event in those diagnosed as having known ischaemic heart disease. However, it is noteworthy that 80 per cent of myocardial events occur in those without a previous diagnosis of coronary disease.

The INTERHEART study assessed the importance of risk factors for coronary artery disease worldwide (Yusuf *et al.* 2004). Investigators around the globe conducted a standardized, case-controlled study involving 30,000 participants in 52 countries. Overall analysis included 12,461 MI patients and 14,637 controls; 76 per cent of cardiac patients were male. The median age for first acute MI was 9 years earlier in men than in women, and 10 per cent of men with an acute MI in the Middle East, Africa, and South Asia were under 40 years of age.

The nine risk factors measured in INTERHEART were smoking, hypertension, diabetes, abdominal obesity, psychosocial factors, consumption of fruits and vegetables, exercise, alcohol consumption, and the ratio of apolipoprotein B (ApoB) to apolipoprotein A (ApoAI). Nine measured and potentially modifiable risk factors accounted for more than 90 per cent of the proportion of the risk for acute MI. Smoking, history of hypertension or diabetes, waist/hip ratio, dietary pattern, lack of physical activity, excess alcohol consumption, blood apolipoproteins, and psychosocial factors were identified as the key risk factors. The effect of these risk factors was consistent in men and women across different geographic regions and by ethnic group. The British Regional Heart Study also found that smoking, blood pressure, and cholesterol accounted for 90 per cent of attributable risk of coronary heart disease (Emberson *et al.* 2003).

1.3 **Outcomes**

Patients with acute coronary syndromes continue to have a poor outcome despite advances in modern therapies. In those admitted with presumed acute coronary syndrome, 36 per cent will ultimately be diagnosed with MI during their index admission (Carruthers *et al.* 2005). The 30-day and 6-month mortality for patients with acute coronary syndrome is particularly high in those with elevated troponin concentrations but is also elevated in those patients with unstable angina who are troponin negative. The presence of ST segment deviation is a stronger predictor of an adverse outcome than elevations in troponin concentrations (Granger *et al.* 2003, Eagle *et al.* 2004). Additionally, more people die in the UK in winter from coronary heart disease: in 2004 to 2005, during the months of winter about 19 per cent more deaths occurred than were expected on the basis of underlying mortality throughout the year. This winter mortality is greater for the elderly, with the winter mortality being over twice as high for the over-85-year-olds as for those over 65 years (British Heart Foundation 2007).

The GRACE registry is the largest multinational cohort of patients covering the full spectrum of acute coronary syndromes. It has inpatient and 6-month follow-up and includes a full spectrum of hospitals and facilities, with 245 hospitals in 30 countries contributing data on about 100,000 patients. Each center reports on the findings and outcomes of the first 10–20 patients with acute coronary disease who present per month. Analysis shows that 34 per cent of presenting patients had ST elevation infarction, 29 per cent had unstable angina, and 30 per cent had experienced non-ST elevation infarction. The remainder had other diagnoses. Eight per cent of patients with ST elevation infarction died as inpatients and 4 per cent of those with non-ST elevation infarction died in the hospital. Patients with unstable angina are confirmed to have a threatening outcome too, with 3 per cent of these patients dying as inpatients. Older age signifies a greater risk, with 10.7 per cent of patients over age 75 with acute coronary disease dying as inpatients compared with 5.6 per cent of those aged between 65 and 75 years. Patients who might be thought to be at low risk, presenting with acute coronary disease but without troponin release or dynamic electrocardiogram (ECG) change, do not have a benign outcome: at 6 months 23 per cent require readmission, 12 per cent have been revascularized, and 3 per cent will have died. Nine factors independently predicted death and the combined end point of death or MI in the period from admission to six months after discharge: age, development (or history) of heart failure, peripheral vascular disease, systolic blood pressure, Killip class, initial serum creatinine concentration, elevated initial cardiac markers, cardiac arrest on admission, and ST segment deviation. The simplified model was robust, with prospectively validated C-statistics of 0.81 for predicting death and 0.73 for death or MI from admission to six months after discharge (Fox *et al*. 2006).

1.4 **Risk scoring tools**

The risk of coronary disease can now be calculated with some confidence using established tools; risk-scoring systems for predicting cardiovascular disease have been devised for use in clinical practice, the majority of which are based on the American Framingham study (Dawber *et al*. 1951).

The Framingham score has been shown to overestimate the actual observed coronary risk in a cohort as a whole, and it seriously underestimated the large gradient in risk by socioeconomic status, particularly in women (SIGN guideline 1997).

The ASSIGN score (ASsessing cardiovascular risk using SIGN guidelines to ASSIGN preventive treatment) has been developed: ASSIGN uses similar classic risk factors to Framingham, but it includes a score for residential postcode as a surrogate for a deprivation index. It also includes family history of cardiovascular disease, defined as coronary disease or stroke in parents or siblings below age 60 or in several close relatives. Results from ASSIGN are similar to those from the Framingham cardiovascular score in many respects but the overall estimation of ten year cardiovascular risk is lower, consistent with some overestimation in the Framingham score. ASSIGN tends to classify more people with a positive family history and who are socially deprived as being at high risk. When used in its own host population it abolished a large social gradient in future cardiovascular victims not identified for preventive treatment by the Framingham cardiovascular score. It therefore improved social equity, although overall discrimination of future events was not greatly improved (Woodward et al. 2007).

QRISK is another risk assessment tool that has been validated against the Framingham cardiovascular disease algorithm: the derivation cohort was 1.28 million patients who were free of diabetes and coronary disease at enrollment. Again the Framingham score overestimated cardiovascular disease risk (at 10 years by 35 per cent): for 2005, UK estimates based on QRISK predicted 3.2 million patients aged 35–74 at high risk, with the Framingham score predicting 4.7 million patients. QRISK and ASSIGN demonstrate that they are more equitable tools in identifying high-risk patients on the basis of social deprivation.

These tools allow for evidence-based decisions to be made regarding who should receive primary preventative therapy that is likely to be of clinical benefit and that is affordable to society.

Key References

British Heart Foundation. (2007) *Coronary Heart Disease statistics*. http://www.heartstats.org (accessed 19/12/2007).

Carruthers KF, Dabbous OH, Flather MD, Starkey I, Jacob A, Macleod D, et al. (2005) Contemporary management of acute coronary syndromes: does the practice match the evidence? The global registry of acute coronary events (GRACE). *Heart* **9**(3): 290–298.

Dawber TR, Meadors GF, Moore FEJ. (1951) Epidemiological approaches to heart disease: the Framingham study. *Am J Public Health* **41**: 279–286.

Eagle KA, Lim MJ, Dabbous OH, Pieper KS, Goldberg RJ, Van de Werf F, et al. (2004) A validated prediction model for all forms of acute coronary syndrome: estimating the risk of 6-month postdischarge death in an international registry. *JAMA* **29**(22): 2727–2733.

Emberson JR, Whincup PH, Morris RW, Walker M. (2003) Re-assessing the contribution of serum total cholesterol, blood pressure and cigarette smoking to the aetiology of coronary heart disease: impact of regression dilution bias. *Eur Heart J* **24**(9): 79–126.

Fox KAA, Dabbous OH, Goldberg, RJ, Pieper KS, Eagle KA, Van de Werf F et al. (2006) Prediction of risk of death and myocardial infarction in the six months after presentation with acute coronary syndrome: prospective multinational observational study (GRACE). *BMJ* **333**: 1091–1094.

Granger CB, Goldberg RJ, Dabbous O, Pieper KS, Eagle KA, Cannon CP, et al. Predictors of hospital mortality in the global registry of acute coronary events. *Arch Intern Med* **3**(9): 2345–2353.

Pais P, Pogue J, Gerstein H, Zachariah E, Savitha D, et al. (1996) Risk factors for acute myocardial infarction in Indians: a case-control study. *Lancet* **348**: 358–363.

SIGN guideline. (1997) Risk estimation and the prevention of cardiovascular disease. http:// www.sign.ac.uk (accessed 19/12/2007)

Sen K, Bonita R. (2000) Global health status: two steps forward, one step back. *Lancet* **356**: 577–582.

Unal B, Critchley JA, Capewell S. (2004) Explaining the decline in coronary heart disease mortality in England and Wales between 1981 and 2000. *Circulation* **109**: 1101–1107.

Woodward M, Brindle P, Tunstall-Pedoe H for the SIGN group on risk estimation. (2007) Adding social deprivation and family history to cardiovascular risk assessment: the ASSIGN score from the Scottish Heart Health Extended Cohort (SHHEC). *Heart* **93**: 172–176.

Yusuf S, Hawken S, Ounpuu S, Dans T, Avezum A, et al. (2004) Effect of potentially modifiable risk factors associated with myocardial infarction in 52 countries (the INTERHEART study): case-control study. *Lancet* **364**: 937–952.

Yusuf S, Hawken S, Ounpuu S, Dans T, Avezum A, Lanas F, et al. (2004) Effect of potentially modifiable risk factors associated with myocardial infarction in 52 countries (the INTERHEART study): case-control study. *Lancet* **364**(9438): 937–952.

Chapter 2

Pathophysiology of acute coronary syndromes

Patrick Calvert and Martin Bennett

> **Key points**
> - Myocardial infarction is caused by plaque rupture and erosion.
> - Most culprit plaques are less than 70 per cent stenosis.
> - Plaque composition and morphology determine clinical effects rather than plaque size.
> - Systemic therapy, for example via cholesterol reduction, alters plaque composition to a more stable morphology.

2.1 Introduction

Myocardial infarction (MI) is predominantly caused by rupture and subsequent vessel thrombosis of high-risk ('vulnerable') plaques in coronary arteries. However, plaque size does not predict behaviour, as most culprit lesions are less than 70 per cent stenosis. In contrast, plaque composition determines outcome, and MIs are particularly associated with thin-cap fibroatheromata (TCFA), where a thin fibrous cap separates a lipid core from the lumen. Unstable plaques typically have a lower fibrous content, a thinner fibrous cap, and a higher lipid content and necrotic core than stable lesions. Changing composition, for example by cholesterol-lowering drugs, is associated with a significant reduction in clinical events, even in the absence of measurable changes in plaque volume.

2.2 Atherosclerotic plaque structure

Atherosclerotic plaques consist of an accumulation of vascular smooth muscle cells (VSMCs), inflammatory cells (macrophages, T-lymphocytes, dendritic cells, and mast cells) underlying a dysfunctional endothelium, together with extracellular lipid, collagen, and matrix (Figure 2.1). These cellular and acellular components are arranged into defined structures within the plaque. Thus, many advanced plaques comprise a VSMC-rich fibrous cap overlying a lipid- and macrophage-rich necrotic core (Figures 2.1 and 2.2). Most atherosclerosis is clinically silent, and consequences of atherosclerosis rarely occur before the development of advanced lesions. This transition from silent to clinically manifest represents profound changes in the components and structure of the plaque, resulting in plaque erosion or plaque rupture, the major triggers to myocardial infarction.

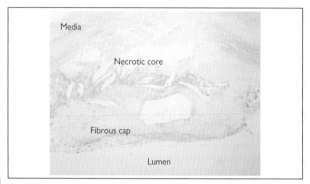

Figure 2.1 Structure of a human atherosclerotic plaque demonstrating a fibrous cap overlying a necrotic core. See also the accompanying colour plate.

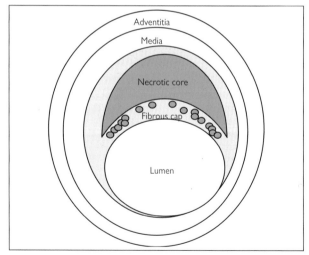

Figure 2.2 Schematic diagram of a fibroatheroma, demonstrating features of a fibrous cap overlying a necrotic core.

Plaque rupture occurs when there is disruption of the fibrous cap, exposing the necrotic core to the blood. The necrotic core is highly thrombogenic, due in major part to the presence of cell-derived microparticles and the presence of tissue factor, which activate thrombin. Local (intraplaque) thrombosis is followed by extension into the lumen, which ultimately may occlude the vessel. In contrast, plaque erosion is defined by the presence of lumen thrombus without an obvious cap rupture into the necrotic core. Compared with plaque rupture, these vessels typically show loss of endothelium over a proteoglycan-rich plaque, and lesser inflammation of an often somewhat smaller, non-calcified lesion. Post-mortem series show that plaque erosion accounts for up to 40 per cent of fatal myocardial infarctions in some patient groups. Erosion is commoner in women than men, and is relatively more frequent in younger than in older patients presenting with MI.

Composition of atherosclerotic plaques determines clinical outcome. Although plaques can show similar structures, there are defining features that determine whether a plaque is more likely to undergo erosion or rupture. These features of stability are important to predict the individual risk and are the major targets for drug therapy for plaque stabilization. Thus, plaques liable to undergo rupture show a thin fibrous cap, a larger necrotic core and lipid component, and a reduced VSMC component than plaques with less likelihood of rupture. The fibrous cap of advanced plaques is thinned from loss of VSMCs, and these thin-cap fibroatheromata are the commonest lesions that rupture. The fibrous caps also typically show macrophage invasion, and there is evidence that macrophages induce cell death of VSMCs and also secrete matrix-degrading enzymes, both of which destabilize the plaque.

Thin-cap fibroatheromata are considered to be the commonest lesion producing plaque rupture. From post-mortem studies, these lesions cluster in the proximal third of the coronary arteries. In particular, recent studies have shown that there are multiple unstable lesions in coronary arteries both upstream and downstream of what is designated the culprit lesion. Lesions are frequently not stenotic, due in part to their small size, and also due to positive (expansile) remodelling, where plaque formation is accompanied by outward expansion of the whole vessel wall, effectively accommodating the growing plaque. Many of the same processes that promote plaque disruption, such as inflammation, haemorrhage, and a lack of fibrous tissue, also promote expansile remodelling, such that the most dangerous lesions are frequently those most easily missed on angiography. Remodelling is mostly seen in proximal vessels, where fibroatheromata cluster, and is often absent in mid or distal vessels, where the same-sized lesions will produce stenosis.

2.3 **Plaque healing and growth**

Although plaque rupture may be fatal, more commonly ruptures are clinically silent. Thus, post-mortem studies demonstrate features of multiple previous ruptures buried within the plaque, with evidence of repair overlying the rupture site. Following rupture, the intraplaque and lumen thrombus is invaded by VSMCs that divide, resorbing and remodelling the thrombus, and replacing it with extracellular matrix and collagen. This sequence of events forms a new fibrous cap over the rupture site. The incorporation and reorganization of thrombus effectively causes plaque growth, as evidenced by studies showing that lumen stenosis is associated with a higher incidence of healed ruptures. Growth of plaques is not linear, but occurs via periods of slow and then rapid growth, as demonstrated by the sudden appearance of new lesions on repeat angiography. It thus follows that plaque repair needs to be as efficient as possible, and any processes that slow repair, for example ongoing inflammation and senescence of VSMCs, can impair the process, predisposing to further plaque rupture.

2.4 **Determination of plaque composition**

Whilst plaque composition is easy to determine *ex vivo*, it is more difficult to identify the different components of plaques *in vivo*. However, an emerging technology may be able to do so, albeit invasively. Radiofrequency intravascular ultrasound (RF-IVUS) uses spectral backscatter of waves emitted from an IVUS catheter to determine the plaque constituents, based upon the different spectral characteristics of fibrous, necrotic core and calcified tissue. Although its spatial resolution is not as good as other techniques for determining anatomy, reported predictive accuracies of 93.5–96.7 per cent when compared to histology have been claimed for RF-IVUS for different plaque components. The catheter is placed in the coronary artery at the time of angiography and motorized pullback gives volume-rendered data of plaque constituents, which are colour-coded. Necrotic core appears red and fibrous material appears dark green (Figure 2.3). The ability of this technique to predict patient outcome is currently being examined in ongoing clinical trials.

2.5 **Treatment to alter plaque composition**

These observations reinforce the concept that changes in plaque composition, rather than plaque volume *per se*, can have profound influences on plaque instability and thus patient risk. We would also predict that therapies aimed at multiple processes that promote plaque instability, or that result in changes in multiple components of

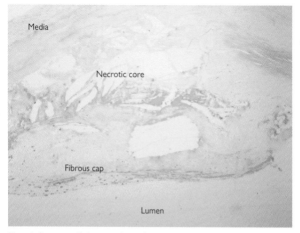

Plate 1 Structure of a human atherosclerotic plaque demonstrating a fibrous cap overlying a necrotic core. Macrophages are identified as brown cells by immunohistochemistry for CD68.

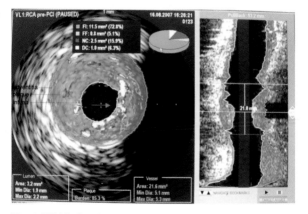

Plate 2 RF-IVUS of a mid-right coronary artery vulnerable plaque that was responsible for an inferior myocardial infarction. Left panel shows axial section, right panel shows longitudinal section of artery with axial section at the white line. There is a pool of necrotic core (red) only separated from the lumen by a cap that is thinner than the axial resolution of RF-IVUS (100 microns). Fibrous tissue is identified by dark green, fibrofatty tissue by light green, necrotic core by red, and calcification by white. Quantification of percentage of each component is as shown.

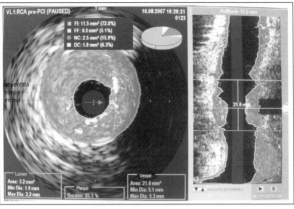

Figure 2.3 RF-IVUS of a mid-right coronary artery vulnerable plaque that was responsible for an inferior myocardial infarction. Left panel shows axial section, right panel shows longitudinal section of artery with axial section at the white line. There is a pool of necrotic core (red) only separated from the lumen by a cap that is thinner than the axial resolution of RF-IVUS (100 microns). Quantification of percentage of each component is as shown. See also the accompanying colour plate.

13

the plaque, would have beneficial effects. For example, statin therapy reduces lipid content of the plaque, reduces macrophage and lymphocyte accumulation and activation, increases VSMC content, increases fibrous cap thickness, and improves endothelial reactivity and function. These effects are all noted at standard therapeutic doses, and in animal models occur without any change in serum cholesterol at all. In contrast, VSMC apoptosis reduces fibrous cap thickness, increases necrotic cores and increases plaque inflammation, all processes predicted to promote plaque instability. This concept may also suggest why there is more limited benefit for agents that target only one process involved in plaque rupture or its consequences. In such a complex process as atherosclerosis it may be that the more 'dirty' the drug, the more processes it affects and the more benefit may be derived.

Plaque repair is also promoted by angioplasty and stenting. Both processes produce a 'controlled' plaque rupture, with tearing of the plaque (including the fibrous cap), dissection into the media, and superficial thrombus formation. Repair of these injured vessels follows the same processes as spontaneous plaque rupture, with resorption of thrombus, VSMC accumulation and matrix formation. Although these latter processes may ultimately produce restenosis or stent stenosis, in most cases the resulting lesion is far more stable than the original plaque.

Key references

Aikawa M, Rabkin E, Okada Y, Voglic SJ, Clinton SK, Brinckerhoff CE, Sukhova GK, Libby P. (1998) Lipid lowering by diet reduces matrix metalloproteinase activity and increases collagen content of rabbit atheroma: a potential mechanism of lesion stabilization. *Circulation* **97**(24): 2433–2444.

Aikawa M, Rabkin E, Voglic SJ, Shing H, Nagai R, Schoen FJ, Libby P. (1998) Lipid lowering promotes accumulation of mature smooth muscle cells expressing smooth muscle myosin heavy chain isoforms in rabbit atheroma. *Circ Res* **83**(10): 1015–1026.

Arbustini E, Dal Bello B, Morbini P, Burke AP, Bocciarelli M, Specchia G, Virmani R. (1999) Plaque erosion is a major substrate for coronary thrombosis in acute myocardial infarction. *Heart* **82**(3): 269–272.

Braganza DM, Bennett MR. (2001) New insights into atherosclerotic plaque rupture. *Postgrad Med J* **77**: 94–98.

Burke AP, Kolodgie FD, Farb A, Weber D, Virmani R. (2002) Morphological predictors of arterial remodeling in coronary atherosclerosis. *Circulation* **105**(3): 297–303.

Burke AP, Kolodgie FD, Farb A, Weber DK, Malcom GT, Smialek J, Virmani R. (2001) Healed plaque ruptures and sudden coronary death: evidence that subclinical rupture has a role in plaque progression. *Circulation* **103**(7): 934–940.

Casscells W, Naghavi M, Willerson JT. (2003) Vulnerable atherosclerotic plaque: a multifocal disease. *Circulation* **107**(16): 2072–2075.

Clarke MC, Figg N, Maguire JJ, Davenport AP, Goddard M, Littlewood TD, Bennett MR. (2006) Apoptosis of vascular smooth muscle cells induces features of plaque vulnerability in atherosclerosis. *Nat Med* **12**(9): 1075–1080.

Crisby M, Nordin-Fredriksson G, Shah PK, Yano J, Zhu J, Nilsson J. (2001) Pravastatin treatment increases collagen content and decreases lipid content, inflammation, metalloproteinases, and cell death in human carotid plaques: implications for plaque stabilization. *Circulation* **103**(7): 926–933.

Davies M, Richardson P, Woolf N, Katz D, Mann J. (1993) Risk of thrombosis in human atherosclerotic plaques: role of extracellular lipid, macrophages, and smooth muscle cell content. *Heart* **69**: 377–381.

Falk E. (1992) Why do plaques rupture? *Circulation* **86**: 11130–11142.

Farb A, Burke AP, Tang AL, Liang TY, Mannan P, Smialek J, Virmani R. (1996) Coronary plaque erosion without rupture into a lipid core. A frequent cause of coronary thrombosis in sudden coronary death. *Circulation* **93**(7): 1354–1363.

Virmani R, Kolodgie FD, Burke AP, Farb A, Schwartz SM. (2000) Lessons from sudden coronary death: a comprehensive morphological classification scheme for atherosclerotic lesions. *Arterioscler Thromb Vasc Biol* **20**(5): 1262–1275.

Williams JK, Sukhova GK, Herrington DM, Libby P. (1998) Pravastatin has cholesterol-lowering independent effects on the artery wall of atherosclerotic monkeys. *J Am Coll Cardiol* **31**: 684–691.

Chapter 3

Prevention of acute coronary syndromes

Anthony S. Wierzbicki

> **Key points**
> - Evaluate cardiovascular risk factors.
> - Intervene on lifestyle-related cardiovascular risk factors: smoking, obesity, etc.
> - Optimize lipid profile and especially maintain low-density lipoprotein-cholesterol (LDL-C) <2 mmol/L.
> - Optimize blood pressure management.
> - Optimize glycaemic control in diabetes.

3.1 Introduction

The epidemiology of cardiovascular disease has been extensively studied over the last 50 years. A number of factors have been shown to be consistently associated with the risk of developing unstable angina and myocardial infarction, which are now subsumed within the term 'acute coronary syndromes'. These include non-modifiable risk factors such as age and gender and a variety of modifiable risk factors including smoking, diabetes, systolic blood pressure, and lipids (Table 3.1). All of these were identified in Caucasian populations in early studies such as the Framingham Heart Study and confirmed in their descendant studies. More recently the data have been generalized to the whole world through the cross-sectional INTERHEART study, which showed that 85–90 per cent of population attributable risk for coronary heart disease was due to 9 factors, including lipids (apolipoprotein B: AI ratio), an apoprotein surrogate for total: high-density lipoprotein-cholesterol (HDL-C), hypertension, smoking, diabetes, abdominal obesity, fruit and vegetable intake, lack of exercise, excess alcohol, and depression (Table 3.2). Other risk factors, though well known and often of similar ancient pedigree, are less often considered, e.g. impaired renal function and microalbuminuria.

Table 3.1 Principal risk factors for atherosclerosis	
Non-modifiable risk factors	**Modifiable risk factors**
Age	Blood pressure
Gender	Total: LDL-cholesterol (apolipoprotein B-100)
	HDL-cholesterol (apolipoprotein A-I)
	Triglycerides
	Blood pressure
	Left ventricular hypertrophy
	Renal function (glomerular filtration rate)
	Glucose
	Insulin
	Microalbuminuria
	Obesity (especially central obesity)
	Inflammation/autoimmune disease

Table 3.2 Risk factors associated with coronary heart disease events in 50 countries in the INTERHEART study			
Risk factor	**% cases**	**% controls**	**Population attributable risk**
Apoliporotein B: AI (quintile extremes)	20.0	33.5	49.2
Smoking	26.8	45.2	35.7
Diabetes	7.5	18.5	9.9
Hypertension	21.9	39	17.9
Central obesity (tertile extremes)	33.3	46.3	20.1
Psychosocial factors	—	—	32.5
Fruit and vegetable intake	42.4	35.8	13.7
Exercise	19.3	14.3	12.2
Alcohol intake	24.5	24.0	6.7
Total risk factors	—	—	90.4
Reproduced from Yusuf et al. (2004).			

3.2 Identification of high-risk patients

The strength of these associations has led to the development of cardiovascular risk calculators in the form of both tables and computerized risk algorithms to convert population-derived data into risk for the individual patient. This approach, though commonly used and recommended in all major guidelines, is only an approximation and it should be remembered that multiple risk determinations are required to derive even approximate values (Figure 3.1). Also many risk factor algorithms are based on historical data or on studies that contained few patients with high-risk conditions (e.g. diabetes) so they may over- or underestimate risk in today's population with a significantly different risk factor burden. Generally all major guidelines recommend pharmacological treatment of risk factors at a cardiovascular risk of 20 per cent/decade. This is approximated by multiplying coronary heart disease risk by 1.3 rather than by specifically considering adding the subtly different risk factor profile for stroke. Many guidelines also recommend the interpolation of missing data by insertion of age- and sex-specific averages or suggest pre-screening by commonly collected variables prior to measurement of lipid or glucose-related risk. Both these approaches introduce significant bias.

Given the unreliability of the risk estimates for patients in the 'grey zone' of 15–25 per cent risk, more specific secondary tests are often used in some countries. Many of these claim to add additional diagnostic value by direct measurement of burden of atherosclerotic disease. Common methods include measurement of carotid intima-media thickness, pulse wave characteristics, endothelial function or plaque burden through assessment of coronary calcium scores. Few of these additional modalities have been convincingly validated in rigorously designed studies powered for comparison of methods by receiver-characteristic curve analysis or by assessment of 'C' statistics. Thus their value to date remains uncertain and their use is not routinely advised in guideline statements.

3.3 **Interventions to prevent acute coronary syndromes**

3.3.1 **Lifestyle measures**

3.3.1.1 *Diet*

Diet contributes to coronary heart disease through its effects on blood pressure and lipids as well as weight (see below). Salt intake has long been suggested to contribute to the burden of hypertension (and indirectly renal impairment) but the data still remain controversial as large-scale epidemiological studies are often confounded by the degree of excess sodium intake in all populations studied to date. Saturated fat contributes to cholesterol levels and obesity as it is metabolized to acetyl-CoA, which can then be used to synthesize triglyceride for storage in adipose tissue or as the basis for cholesterol production in the liver. Studies of rural populations have shown

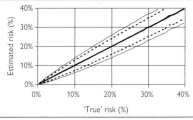

Figure 3.1 Relationship between measured and 'true' risk for the Framingham risk equation (1991 version). Confidence interval based on single (---) or triplicate (-) determinations

a direct correlation between plasma cholesterol levels and coronary heart disease rates in different populations but with subtle differences in slopes (Figure 3.1). The differences have been attributed to the role of other factors, including the poly- and mono-unsaturated fatty acids present in high quantities in the Mediterranean diet. There is evidence on lipid surrogates that diets reduced in salt and saturated fat and increased in polyunsaturates reduce blood pressure and cholesterol levels, and diets such as that from the Diet And Sodium in Hypertension (DASH) study are recommended for patients at risk of coronary heart disease (CHD). There are no endpoint studies of the effects of diet that have been positive; the Multiple Risk Factor Intervention Trial (MRFIT) failed to show much difference in either risk factors or events at 6 years despite recruiting 14,866 patients. Endpoint evidence for other diets is rarer and controversial. A Mediterranean diet in the Lyon Heart Health Study reduced cardiovascular events by 50–70 per cent in an underpowered study, while the prescription of oily fish (mackerel) in the DART study reduced mortality in the initial study by 29 per cent but increased events in a highly confounded follow-up study (DART-2).

3.3.1.2 *Exercise*

Exercise is recommended for all patients at risk of CHD. Again, the amount and intensity are controversial. It seems that more than 30 minutes a day of moderately strenuous aerobic exercise reduces CHD events in both epidemiological and some intervention studies. Further increases in intensity and time may offer extra benefits. Exercise both reduces the amount of adipose tissue, especially visceral adipose tissue, and increases muscle insulin sensitivity. It has benefits on multiple aspects of the metabolic syndrome (Table 3.3), a constellation of risk factors associated with increased risk of CHD and especially

Figure 3.1 is reproduced with permission from Reynolds TM, Twomey P, Wierzbicki AS. (2002). Accuracy of cardiovascular risk estimation in patients without diabetes. *J Cardiovasc Risk*, **9**: 183–90.

Table 3.3 Principal definitions of the metabolic syndrome

Risk factor	National Cholesterol Education Program (NCEP)	International Diabetes Federation (IDF)
Waist circumference (cm)	Caucasians Male >102 Female >88	Caucasians USA: Male >102, female >88 Europe: Male >94, female >80
HDL-cholesterol (mmol/L)	Male <1.0 Female <1.2	Male <1.0, female <1.2 or HDL-raising therapy
Triglycerides (mmol/L)	>1.7	>1.7 or TG-lowering therapy
Blood pressure (mmHg)	>130/85	>130/85 or anti-hypertensive therapy
Fasting glucose (mmol/L)	>6.1, now >5.6	>5.6 or established diabetes
Method	Any 3	Abdominal obesity and any 2 others

Based on NCEP (2001) and IDF (2005).

Type 2 diabetes (Figure 3.2). There is, however, a clear relationship between rigorous exercise and diet advice and the prevention of progression of impaired fasting glucose/impaired glucose tolerance to frank Type 2 diabetes, as shown by the 54–58 per cent reduction in new cases in the Finnish and US Diabetes Prevention Programs. It is assumed by implication that a reduction in cardiovascular risk will follow from this, though no studies have yet been specifically designed to test this endpoint in patients with the metabolic syndrome.

3.3.1.3 Alcohol

The relationship between alcohol and CHD is complex. Epidemiology shows a J-shaped curve, with increased risk for teetotallers and also for individuals consuming excessive amounts of alcohol, though the exact cut-off for this is controversial. In general a moderate alcohol intake (<20 units/week in a male, <15 units/week in a female) is associated with a reduction in cardiovascular disease in epidemiological studies. There are no intervention studies in this field.

3.3.1.4 Weight reduction

Obesity is a long-established cardiovascular risk factor and excessive body mass index (BMI) (clinical obesity >30 kg/m^2) has long been associated with CHD risk. More recently the limitations of BMI measurement, particularly with regard to distinguishing 'heavy' muscle

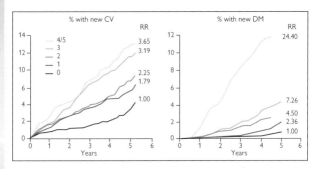

Figure 3.2 Occurrence of cardiovascular events (CV) and new diabetes mellitus (DM) in middle-aged men from the West of Scotland Coronary Outcomes Prevention Study. 26.2 per cent had 'NCEP-defined' metabolic syndrome; CHD event rate in DM = 17.6 per cent. RR = relative risk.

from 'light' fat, have been noticed and the excess risk associated with visceral adipose tissue has been noted. Thus increasingly waist circumference is replacing BMI in many risk identification programmes, though the diversity of body habitus means that different waist cut-offs for assessment of metabolic syndrome risk have to be used in different ethnic groups. In the morbidly obese, other weight-associated complications including sleep apnoea increase risk of cardiovascular disease further. Few studies have assessed how weight reduction may affect cardiovascular risk. In the morbidly obese (BMI >40 kg/m^2) registry studies show a 75 per cent reduction in diabetes and a 35 per cent reduction in total mortality with bariatric surgery. In moderately obese patients recruited to the Xenical (XENDOS) study, orlistat therapy was associated with a 2.8 kg weight loss and a 37 per cent reduction in cases of new Type 2 diabetes. Outcome trials on cardiovascular events with agents that produce an average 4.5–5 kg (per cent) weight loss as opposed to the average 2.7 kg (3 per cent) seen with orlistat are underway with sibutramine (SCOUT) and rimonabant (CRESCENDO).

3.3.1.5 *Smoking cessation*
Smoking cessation is associated with lower rates of coronary events, with about a 30 per cent reduction in events in the first year and virtually complete benefit seen after 7 years cessation. Many patients quit immediately after an event but unfortunately many later relapse so that rates are often little reduced at one year. A multiplicity of methods are available for smoking cessation though many have a poor evidence base. Willpower and hypnosis have a quit rate of

Figure 3.2. is reproduced with permission from Sattar N, Gaw A, Scherbakova O, *et al.* (2003). Metabolic syndrome with and without C-reactive protein as a predictor of coronary heart disease and diabetes in the West of Scotland Coronary Prevention Study. *Circulation*, **108**: 414–19.

about 9 per cent, while nicotine replacement therapy increases this to about 17 per cent over 4 weeks. Data from large-scale studies comparing different forms of nicotine replacement therapy are rare. A number of drug therapies exist to reduce cravings and do increase quit rates when included in a tailored smoking cessation programme. In one trial with a carbon monoxide-confirmed 1-year endpoint the placebo quit rate was 4.9 per cent, bupropion had a 6.5 per cent quit rate, and the nicotinic acid alpha-4 receptor partial agonist varenicline was associated with a 14.4 per cent quit rate. There are no prospective outcome studies that have compared methods of smoking cessation for their benefits on CHD events.

3.3.2 **Direct risk factor interventions**

3.3.2.1 *Aspirin and anti-platelet agents*

Currently it is impossible to measure thrombosis risk in a systematic reproducible manner, though claims are made for the benefits of assessing urinary thromboxane B_2 levels. The mainstay of therapy is aspirin 75/81 mg, which was shown to reduce cardiovascular events in the ISIS-2 trial. The Anti-Platelet Triallists' Collaboration has shown that aspirin therapy is associated with a 32 per cent risk reduction and studies in primary monotherapy prevention show benefits in men from age 40 and women from age 55. Dipyridamole showed no benefits on CHD events but has been shown to be useful when added to aspirin for the purpose of stroke prevention in the ESPRIT study. Clopidogrel showed equivalent cardiovascular benefits to aspirin in the secondary prevention CAPRIE study, with the suggestion of extra benefit in patients with peripheral arterial disease. Despite benefits of aspirin combined with clopidogrel therapy in the acute management of acute coronary syndromes in the CURE study, the combination of aspirin and clopidogrel showed no benefit over aspirin monotherapy and an increase in haemorrhagic events in the CHARISMA trial.

3.3.2.2 *Reducing LDL-cholesterol*

The evidence linking LDL-cholesterol (LDL-C) reduction with reductions in CHD rates is vast and compelling and many studies have been specifically performed in patients with acute coronary syndromes. The original studies using cholestyramine (Lipids Research Clinics) or partial ileal bypass surgery (Program on Surgical Correction of Hyperlipidemia) showed a 18–34 per cent reduction in CHD events but no benefit on mortality. The landmark Scandinavian Simvastatin Survival Study (4S) showed a 34 per cent reduction in CHD events, allied to a 30 per cent reduction in mortality in patients with stable coronary disease. These data were later extended to acute coronary syndromes in the Lipid Intervention with Pravastatin in Ischemic Disease study, where pravastatin 40 mg reduced events by 25 per cent. In the underpowered MIRACL study, 80 mg od atorvastatin achieving a LDL-cholesterol of 1.9 mmol/L and a 52 per cent LDL-C reduction demonstrated a 16 per cent reduction in CHD events (including angina) against placebo in patients with acute coronary syndrome being managed medically. Later trials accepted the results from the Heart Protection Study, which showed a 24 per cent benefit with prescription of 40 mg simvastatin and did not have placebo arms. The data for reducing LDL-C with statins are summarized in the Cholesterol Treatment Triallists' collaborative project, which shows a 12 per cent reduction in mortality and 22 per cent reduction in CHD events per 1 mmol/L LDL-C reduction. The PROVE-IT study compared 40 mg pravastatin with 80 mg atorvastatin in a non-inferiority design but demonstrated that the extra 0.86 mmol/L reduction in LDL-C was associated with a significant further 16 per cent reduction in CHD events in patients with acute coronary syndromes. In *post hoc* sub-group analysis benefits were seen in patients with LDL-C < 1.5 mmol/L, with no significant excess of adverse events. In contrast, in the more complex design of the 'Z' arm of the Aggrastat to Zocor (A-Z) trial, placebo/40 mg simvastatin was only slightly (and non-significantly) inferior to 40/80 mg simvastatin, with an 11 per cent excess of events and a net difference of 0.4 mmol/L between the 2 arms. Meta-analysis of these trials is complex but suggests there is benefit to achieving a LDL-C in the range 1.75–2.00 mmol/L in patients with acute coronary syndromes.

3.3.2.3 *Optimization of general lipid profiles*
Few data are specifically available in acute coronary syndromes for other lipid-lowering agents. Fibrates reduce triglycerides and increase lipoprotein particle sizes and may raise HDL-C and reduce LDL-C in some cases. In primary prevention gemfibrozil therapy in the Helsinki Heart Study was associated with a 23 per cent reduction in coronary events but not mortality, while in a secondary prevention population with low HDL-C (<0.95 mmol/L) and not receiving statin therapy its use was associated with a 24 per cent reduction in cardiovascular disease events in the Veterans Administration HDL Intervention Trial. In contrast, in the secondary prevention World Health Organization Clofibrate trial and later in the Coronary Drug Project, clofibrate reduced events by 18–20 per cent but increased mortality by 8 per cent. In a mixed group of patients with Type 2 diabetes fenofibrate therapy was associated with an 11 per cent reduction in cardiovascular disease events and a non-significant 11 per cent reduction in CHD events, with the benefits being seen surprisingly in patients in primary prevention or not receiving statin therapy. Meta-analysis suggests that fibrates may have beneficial effects in non-fatal myocardial infarction or interventional procedures but not on stroke or mortality. They thus remain second-line agents until the combination fibrate–statin study in diabetes (ACCORD) reports.

Niacin increases HDL-C by up to 30 per cent and reduces LDL-C and triglycerides. It showed a 23 per cent reduction in CHD events in the Coronary Drug project and at 6.2 and 15 years shows a reduction in cardiovascular mortality. Its use has been limited by its prostaglandin D_2-related flushing and reports of hyperglycaemia. Newer preparations have reduced rates of flushing and further optimization is underway. When added to statins niacin reduces the progression of atherosclerosis in carotid and coronary arteries and may reduce events, as shown in the Familial Atherosclerosis Treatment Study follow-up. Large-scale studies combining niacin with optimal statin therapy in patients with established CHD and dyslipidaemia (AIM-HIGH) or in high-risk patients Heart Protection-2 (HPS-2) are underway.

Synthetic/extracted omega-3 fatty acids have also been assessed in CHD. In the GISSI-P open-label study using a dose of 1 g Omacr® (460 mg eicosapentaenoic acid and 380 mg docosahexaenoic acids), omega-3 fatty acid therapy reduced CHD events by 10–15 per cent, with a 40 per cent benefit seen in the first 3 months and in patients with acute coronary syndromes without any significant effect on lipid profiles. More recently the JELIS study of 1.8 g eicosapentenoic acid added to pravastatin therapy reduced CHD events by 19 per cent in a slightly different set of sub-groups. At higher doses omega-3 fatty acids reduce triglyceride concentrations but no endpoint studies have investigated the utility if high doses of omega-3 fatty acid therapy in acute coronary syndromes.

3.3.2.4 *Optimization of glycaemic control*

Patients with diabetes have increased rates of CHD and after 7–15 years of diabetes their cardiovascular disease risk becomes equivalent to that of normoglycaemic patients with established CHD. Many guidelines consider all patients with diabetes to be CHD-risk equivalents but others suggest risk calculation based on specific risk factor profiles (e.g. UK Prospective Diabetes Survey [UKPDS] algorithm). There are few data on Type 1 diabetes though the rates of cardiovascular disease are vastly increased. In the Diabetes Care and Control Trial (DCCT) increased progression of carotid intima–media thickness was associated with age, smoking, blood pressure, glycaemic control, microalbuminuria, and with lipids having a weak role. In contrast, in Type 2 diabetes risks of macrovascular events are associated with LDL-C and HDL-C to a greater extent. The role of optimizing glucose control in Type 2 diabetes was investigated in UKPDS and improved glycaemic control was associated with a 15 per cent reduction in CHD events. In obese patients receiving metformin a 34 per cent reduction was observed and controversial data were found about sulphonylureas (a 58 per cent increase in CHD events in a small sub-study). In actual fact it seems that sulphonylureas have little adverse effect and general better glycaemic control is associated with moderate benefits on CVD risk. This is being further investigated as part of the glucose arm of the ACCORD study.

More recently, thiazolidinediones (glitazones) have been introduced. The only pre-specified data that exist on this drug class comprise the use of pioglitazone 45 mg in secondary prevention patients with Type 2 diabetes. In the PROactive study this was associated with a non-significant 10 per cent reduction in CHD events and a borderline significant 16 per cent reduction in cardiovascular disease events at the cost of an increase in heart failure. Meta-analysis of the data from phase 3 studies, registry studies, and a premature interim analysis of the secondary prevention RECORD study with rosiglitazone, which has less beneficial lipid actions, has suggested it may increase CHD events by up to 43 per cent as far as confirming increased rates of cardiac failure.

The role of glitazones in patients with acute coronary syndromes remains unclear but it seems that they may be of only at most marginal benefit and that that benefit may be agent-specific.

3.3.2.5 *Reduction of systolic blood pressure*
The role of blood pressure reduction on cardiovascular events was addressed in the Antihypertensive and Lipid-Lowering Treatment to Prevent Heart Attack Trial (ALLHAT). This trial had a complex design to maintain integrity of the 4 investigational arms (alpha-blocker; angiotensin-converting enzyme inhibitor [ACE-I]; calcium channel blocker [CCB]; and thiazide diuretic) given the need for ancillary therapies (beta-blockers; α-methyldopa; reserpine). This design probably led to the premature demise of the alpha-blocker arm due to increased rates of stroke and cardiac failure as a consequence of inadequate blood pressure control. All the other arms of the study showed similar results indicating that attainment of optimal blood pressure was necessary to reduce cardiovascular events. The actual blood pressure targets are derived from the somewhat flawed Hypertension Optimal Treatment study, which used a diastolic (rather than systolic) blood pressure design and unfortunately achieved almost identical control in all arms. Optimal blood pressures are set at 140/90 mmHg in normoglycaemic patients and 130/85 mmHg in patients with diabetes. Subsequent studies have identified a slight 9 per cent CHD benefit to the use of ACE-I/CCB regimes as opposed to beta-blocker–thiazide in the Anglo-Scandinavian Coronary Outcomes Study (ASCOT) and noted an increase in new cases of diabetes in patients receiving a combination of beta-blocker and thiazide. Data from studies with angiotensin-2 type 1 receptor blockers suggest advantages over beta-blocker–based regimes in the LIFE study in patients with hypertension and left ventricular hypertrophy, but little advantage over CCB-based regimes in secondary prevention patients in the VALUE and VALIANT studies.

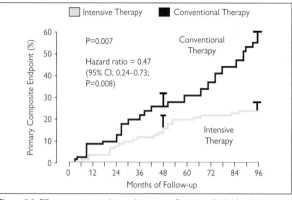

Figure 3.3 Effect on major cardiovascular events of intensive lipid, blood pressure and glycaemic control compared to usual care in patients with type-2 diabetes mellitus. Reproduced with permission from Gaede *et al.* (2003).

In patients with Type 2 diabetes optimization of lipid, glycaemic and blood pressure control led to a 50 per cent reduction in CHD events in the STENO-2 (Figure 3.3), demonstrating the benefits of multiple risk factor optimization in this high-risk group. Further investigation of optimal blood pressure and glycaemic control forms part of the blood pressure arm of ACCORD.

3.4 **Conclusion**

While epidemiological evidence for the association of lifestyle factors with CHD and acute coronary syndromes is strong, there is a lack of properly designed intervention studies in the field. In contrast, as is so often the case, there is extensive evidence from many studies that optimizing LDL-C levels and blood pressure and prescribing aspirin is necessary in all patients, and that improving glycaemic control in patients with diabetes will reduce subsequent cardiovascular events.

Key references

Alberti KG, Zimmet P, Shaw J, and the International Diabetes Federation. (2005) The metabolic syndrome: a new world wide definition. *Lancet* **366**: 1059–1062.

The Antihypertensive and Lipid-Lowering Treatment to Prevent Heart Attack Trial (ALLHAT) Investigators. (2002) Major outcomes in high-risk hypertensive patients randomized to angiotensin-converting enzyme inhibitor or calcium channel blocker vs diuretic: the Antihypertensive and Lipid-Lowering Treatment to Prevent Heart Attack Trial (ALLHAT). *J Am Med Assoc* **288**: 2981–2997.

Anti-Platelet Triallists' Collaboration. (2002) Collaborative meta-analysis of randomised trials of antiplatelet therapy for prevention of death, myocardial infarction, and stroke in high risk patients. *Br Med J* **324**: 71–86.

Cannon CP, Steinberg BA, Murphy SA, Mega JL, Braunwald E. (2006) Meta-analysis of cardiovascular outcomes trials comparing intensive versus moderate statin therapy. *J Am Coll Cardiol* **48**: 438–445.

Gaede P, Vedel P, Larsen N, Jensen GV, Parving HH, Pedersen O. (2003) Multifactorial intervention and cardiovascular disease in patients with type 2 diabetes. *New Engl J Med* **348**(5): 383–393.

National Cholesterol Education Program (NCEP) Expert Panel on Detection, Evaluation, and Treatment of High Blood Cholesterol in Adults (Adult Treatment Panel III). Executive summary of the Third Report. (2001) *J Am Med Assoc* **285**: 2486–2497.

Reynolds TM, Twomey P, Wierzbicki AS, *et al.* (2002) Accuracy of cardiovascular risk estimation in patients without diabetes. *J Cardiovasc Risk* **9**: 183–90.

Sattar N, Gaw A, Scherbakova O, *et al.* (2003) Metabolic syndrome with and without C-reactive protein as a predictor of coronary heart disease and diabetes in the West of Scotland Coronary Prevention Study. *Circulation* **108**: 414–419.

Yusuf S, Hawken S, Ounpuu S, Dans T, Avezum A, Lanas F, McQueen M, Budaj A, Pais P, Varigos J, Lisheng L. (2004) Effect of potentially modifiable risk factors associated with myocardial infarction in 52 countries (the INTERHEART study): case-control study. *Lancet* **364**: 937–952.

Chapter 4

Initial evaluation

Hao Chin and Derek Connolly

> **Key points**
> - Have a low threshold of suspicion as symptoms can be atypical.
> - Early and repeated electro-cardiograms (ECGs) are very helpful.
> - Cardiac biomarkers are increasingly useful for both diagnosis and prognosis.

4.1 Introduction

Angina pectoris was first described by Heberden 200 years ago and the first acute myocardial infarction was documented by Herrick a century later. In the early 1970s, Conti and Fowler introduced the terminology of 'unstable angina' to signify an intermediate diagnosis between the 2 extreme entities of stable angina pectoris and myocardial infarction (MI). In 1985, Fuster coined the phrase 'acute coronary syndrome' (ACS) to highlight the pathophysiological continuum between unstable angina and Q-wave myocardial infarction. Hence with the evolving understanding of the concept of acute coronary syndrome encompassing unstable angina, non-ST–elevation myocardial infarction (NSTEMI) and ST-elevation myocardial infarction (STEMI), prompt and accurate identification of acute coronary syndrome has since become a challenging diagnostic and triaging skill for clinicians in accident and emergency departments.

This chapter reviews the role of history-taking, physical examination, electrocardiogram (ECG) and the use of biomarkers of myocardial necrosis (creatine kinase MB cardioselective isoenzyme, troponin T or I) as an integrated tool to aid diagnosing and triaging patients with ACS.

4.2 Clinical presentation

4.2.1 Angina

In spite of the central hallmark of ACS being chest pain, it remains difficult at times to distinguish between cardiac and non-cardiac pain.

Typical 'ischaemic pain' is described as chest tightness, pressure-like heaviness, an aching feeling or even a constricting sensation around the throat. It is unaffected by respiration, movement or position. Sharp, stabbing or positional pain is less likely to represent ischaemic pain, although this should not be written off as 'musculo-skeletal' pain, as one study showed 22 per cent of patients with such pain turned out to have acute ischaemia. Moreover, 7 per cent of the patients with pain fully reproduced by pressure palpation and 24 per cent of patients with pain partially reproduced by palpation had ischaemia.

Unstable angina has traditionally categorized new-onset angina, increasing angina, rest angina, and recurrent ischaemia after myocardial infarction (Table 4.1). Braunwald has refined this by suggesting a classification of unstable angina based on severity, precipitant, and concurrent anti-anginal therapy (Table 4.2).

Table 4.1 Clinical presentation of ACS

Type of angina	Presentation
New-onset angina	New onset angina of at least CCS class III severity
Rest angina	Angina occurring at rest and prolonged, usually > 20 minutes
Increasing angina ('crescendo' angina)	Angina that has become more frequent, longer in duration or lower in threshold
Early post-MI angina	Recurrent ischaemic chest pain within 30 days after MI

Table 4.2 Braunwald classification of unstable angina

Classification element	Class	Definition
Severity	I	Symptoms with exertion
	II	Symptoms at rest: subacute (2–30 days prior)
	III	Symptoms at rest: acute (within prior 48 hours)
Precipitant	A	Secondary
	B	Primary
	C	Post-infarction
Therapy presented during symptoms	1	No treatment
	2	Usual angina therapy
	3	Maximal therapy

Hence a patient with acute chest pain on minimal exertion or at rest while taking usual medical therapy would be classified as class IIIB$_2$, the most common presentation in the Global Unstable Angina Registry and Treatment Evaluation (GUARANTEE) study.

4.2.2 Angina equivalents

Dyspnoea is regarded as the most significant angina-equivalent symptom, being present in about one-third of patients with infarction in some studies. As a principal complaint, it is more commonly associated with a final diagnosis of non-ACS in one study (18 per cent non-ACS vs 7 per cent ACS; $P \leq 0.001$), suggesting a high prevalence of patients with lung disease in the study population. Yet the finding of 4–14 per cent of MI patients and 5 per cent of unstable angina patients presenting with only sudden dyspnoea highlights the necessity of high clinical suspicion index for ACS.

4.2.3 Atypical presentations

Up to one-third of patients hospitalized for acute MI either presented with no chest pain or had chief complaints other than chest pain (i.e. dyspnoea, extreme fatigue, abdominal discomfort, nausea or syncope). **Diaphoresis** occurs in 20–50 per cent of MI patients and can be the only presenting symptoms in patients with ACS, and **vomiting** is also very common in ACS.

4.3 Physical findings

In comparison with symptomatology of ACS and ECG findings, physical examination is generally less informative in diagnosing ACS. The physical examination may be unremarkable but Box 4.1 illustrates possible examination findings.

Chest pain partially or fully reproduced by palpation should by no means lure clinicians into a false sense of security, as 11 per cent of patients may have ACS.

Box 4.1 Physical examination findings in ACS

- Pallor, cold peripheries
- Tachycardia
- High respiratory rate
- High systolic blood pressure
- Cardiogenic shock
- S3 gallops
- Basilar rales/crepitations

4.4 **Electrocardiogram**

An urgent ECG on anyone with a potential ACS leads to prompt diagnosis and appropriate treatment. A finding of ST-segment elevation or the presence of new left bundle branch block may suggest ST-elevation myocardial infarction. Untreated, most ST-segment elevation will eventually evolve to a Q-wave myocardial infarction. On the other hand, most non-ST elevation ACS will either be diagnosed as unstable angina or non-ST–segment elevation MI based on the absence or presence of various biomarkers (commonly troponin T or I) for myocardial necrosis (see Figure 4.1).

ST-segment deviation and T-wave changes has long been regarded as the *sine qua non* of ECG diagnosis of ACS. **ST-depression** signifies 'subendocardial ischaemia', and its persistence and severity correlates with the probability of myocardial infarction. About 50–67 per cent of patients with new or presumed new isolated ST-segment depression have infarctions, although differential diagnoses of hyperventilation, uptake of digoxin, hypokalaemia, and left ventricular strain should be considered.

Inverted T-waves may reflect acute ischaemia, albeit a lower risk of ischaemia compared to ST-deviation. This ECG change was shown by one study to account for 10 per cent of coronary care unit (CCU) admissions, of whom 22 per cent had acute MI. Differential diagnoses of isolated T-wave changes include prior myocardial damage or left ventricular strain.

Q-waves can be diagnostic of myocardial infarction as shown by the MILIS study, in which isolated new or presumed new inferior or anterior Q-waves were associated with 51 per cent and 77 per cent of corresponding acute infarctions. However, the same study also showed 12 per cent of healthy young male have inferior Q-waves. Isolated Q-waves should not be used to identify ACS since it rarely manifests in acute MI and may even be absent altogether.

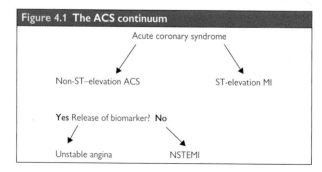

Figure 4.1 The ACS continuum

Acute coronary syndrome

Non-ST–elevation ACS   ST-elevation MI

Yes Release of biomarker? **No**

Unstable angina   NSTEMI

Normal ECGs should not deter the diagnosis of ACS as 1–6 per cent of patients with such ECGs have been found to have ACS. Although a normal ECG and an atypical history in a patient points to a diagnosis of non-ACS, patients with a normal ECG and a suggestive clinical presentation still have a significant risk of ACS, especially if the ECG was done when the patient was pain-free. In addition, conventional 12-lead ECG is confounded by its incomplete coverage of myocardial activity, especially that of the right ventricle, posterior-basal or lateral walls (i.e. the territory of the circumflex artery).

Given the realization that a normal ECG only represents a brief static representation of the whole picture of ACS, **serial ECGs** are mandatory to look specifically for dynamic ST-T wave changes. In addition, **continuous Holter monitoring** is needed in patients strongly suspected of having ACS, to improve the detection of ST deviation (a sign of ongoing ischaemia) as well as that of arrhythmia, a complication more associated with NSTEMI than with unstable angina. Continuous ST-segment monitoring has been shown in studies to be more sensitive than patients' symptoms in identification of evidence of ischaemia within 24 hours of hospital admission.

4.5 **Biomarkers of myocardial necrosis**

The use of biomarkers (CK-MB, troponin-T or I) has now become an invaluable tool in diagnosing ACS in conjunction with the traditional history-taking, physical examination, and ECG findings. These are used to further categorize ACS patients as NSTEMI (see Figure 4.1). The availability of troponins, being more sensitive and specific than CK-MB, has lent itself to an increased diagnosis of patients with NSTEMI.

The significance of these biomarkers has been shown by numerous studies to extend to the prognostic implications of patients with NSTEMI. Further to the association of positive results with worsened prognosis, there is a linear relationship between the magnitude of release and subsequent mortality. This has led to the concept of risk stratification in the management of ACS.

4.6 **Risk stratification**

ACS, being a pathophysiological and clinical continuum, results in a heterogeneous group of patients presenting to a casualty department. It is therefore understandable that risk stratification is essential amid mounting clinical and economic pressure to aid rapid decision-making and guidance of subsequent patient management. The correlation between the gradient of risk in ACS patients with their prognosis has led to the development of various predictive models. High-risk patients identified by certain clinical features, ECG findings, and/or presence of biomarkers are deemed to have more adverse outcomes (Table 4.3). These patients appear to derive greater benefit from aggressive medical and/or interventional therapy.

The Thrombolysis in myocardial infarction-11B trial has yielded a simplified yet effective model of risk stratification gaining increasing usage. The seven independent predictors identified are shown in Box 4.2.

Table 4.3 Clinical features of high-risk ACS	
Area	**Risk factors**
History	Advanced age (>70 years)
	Diabetes mellitus
	Post-myocardial infarction angina
	Prior peripheral vascular disease
	Prior cerebrovascular disease
Clinical presentation	Acute or subacute rest pain
	Secondary unstable angina
	Heart failure or hypotension; ventricular arrhythmias
ECG	ST-segment deviation ≥ 0.05 mV
	T-wave inversion ≥ 0.3 mV
	Left bundle branch block
Cardiac markers	Increased troponin T or I or CK-MB
	Increased C-reactive protein or white blood cell count
	Increased B-type natriuretic peptide
	Increased CD-40 ligand
	Elevated glucose or haemoglobin A1C; elevated creatinine
Angiogram	Thrombus; three vessel disease; reduced ejection fraction

Box 4.2 Predictors of high risk from the TIMI-11B trial

- Age ≥ 65 years
- $\geq$ three cardiovascular risk factors
- Significant coronary artery stenosis (≥ 50per cent)
- ST-segment deviation
- Severe anginal symptoms
- Use of aspirin in the last 7 days
- Elevated cardiac biomarkers

4.7 **Conclusion**

The continuum of the acute coronary syndrome has provided diagnostic challenge to clinicians facing thousands of patients admitted with acute non-traumatic chest pain yearly. Risk stratification by employing complementary clinical, ECG, and biochemical information has undoubtedly provided much-needed guidance in rapid clinical assessment. The use of myocardial biomarkers, in particular troponins, has increased the diagnostic sensitivity and specificity of ACS. More importantly, it allows both short- and long-term prognostication of patients who have been diagnosed with ACS. This ultimately provides a strong foundation for subsequent evidence-based clinical management of patients with ACS.

Key references

Akkerhuis KM, Klootwijk PA, Lindeboom W et al. (2001) Recurrent ischaemia during continuous multilead ST-segment monitoring identifies patients with acute coronary syndromes at high risk of adverse cardiac events: meta-analysis of three studies involving 995 patients. Eur Heart J 22: 1997–2006.

Alonzo AA, Simon AB, Feilieb M. (1975) Prodromata of myocardial infarction and sudden death. Circulation 52: 1056–1062.

Antman EM, Cohen M, Bernink PJ et al. (2000) The TIMI risk score for unstable angina/non-ST elevation MI: a method for prognostication and therapeutic decision-making. J Am Med Assoc 284: 835–842.

Antman EM, Tanasijevic MJ, Thompson B et al. (1996) Cardiac-specific troponin I levels to predict the risk of mortality in patients with acute coronary syndromes. New Engl J Med 335: 1342.

Behar S, Schor S, Kariv I et al. (1977) Evaluation of electrocardiogram in emergency room as a decision-making tool. Chest 71: 486–491.

Braunwald E. (1989) Unstable angina. A classification. Circulation 80: 410–414.

Conti CR, Greene B, Pitt B, Griffith L, Hymphries O, Brawley R, Taylor D, Bender H, Gott V, Ross RS. (1971) Coronary surgery in unstable angina pectoris. Circulation 44(suppl II): 11–154.

DeWood MA, Stifer WF, Simpson CS et al. (1986) Coronary arteriographic findings soon after non-Q-wave myocardial infarction. New Engl J Med 315: 417–423.

Fowler NO. (1971) Preinfarction angina: a need for an objective definition and for a controlled clinical trial of its management. Circulation 44: 755–758.

Fuster V, Steele PM, Chesebro JH. (1985) Role of platelets and thrombosis in coronary atherosclerotic disease and sudden death. J Am Coll Cardiol 5: 175B–184B.

Goldberger AL. (1979) Myocardial infarction electrocardiographic differential diagnosis, 2nd edn. CV Mosby, St Louis.

Goodman SG, Fitchett D, Armstrong PW et al. (2003) Randomized evaluation of the safety and efficacy of enoxaparin versus unfractionated heparin in high-risk patients with non-ST-segment elevation acute coronary syndromes receiving the glycoprotein IIb/IIIa inhibitor eptifibatide. Circulation 107: 238.

Granborg J, Grande P, Pederson A. (1986) Diagnostic and prognostic significance of transient isolated negative T waves in suspected acute myocardial infarction. Am J Cardiol 57: 203–207.

Hamm CW, Heeschen C, Goldmann B et al for the c7E3 Fab Antiplatelet Therapy in Unstable Refractory Angina (CAPTURE) Study Investigators. (1999) Benefit of abciximab in patients with refractory unstable angina in relation to serum troponin T levels. New Engl J Med 340: 1623.

Heberden W. (1772) Some accounts of a disorder of the breast. Med Trans R Coll Phys Lond.

Heeschen C, Hamm CW, Goldmann B et al for the PRISM Study Investigators. (1999) Troponin concentration for stratification of patients with acute coronary syndromes in relation to therapeutic efficacy of tirofiban. Lancet 354: 1757.

Herrick JB. (1912) Clinical features of sudden obstruction of the coronary arteries. J Am Med Assoc 59: 2015–2020.

Joint European Society of Cardiology/American College of Cardiology Committee. (2000) Myocardial infarction redefined. A consensus document of the Joint European Society of Cardiology/American College of Cardiology committee for the redefinition of myocardial infarction. J Am Coll Cardiol 36: 959.

Kaul P, Newby LK, Fu Y, Hasselblad V, Mahaffey KW, Christenson RH et al for PARAGON-B Investigators. (2003) Troponin T and quantitative ST-segment depression offer complementary prognostic information in the risk stratification of acute coronary syndrome patients. J Am Coll Cardiol 41(3): 371–380.

Kennedy JW. (1986) Non-Q-wave myocardial infarction. New Engl J Med 315: 451–453.

Kinlen LJ. (1973) Incidence and presentation of myocardial infarction in an English community. Br Heart J 35: 616–622.

Kleiman N, Lakkis N, Cannon C et al. (2002) Prospective analysis of creatine kinase muscle-brain fraction and comparison with troponin T to predict cardiac risk and benefit of an invasive strategy in patients with non-ST-elevation acute coronary syndromes. J Am Coll Cardiol 40: 1044.

Lee TH, Cook F, Weisberg M, Sargent RK, Wilson C, Goldman L. (1985) Acute chest pain in the emergency room: identification and examination of low-risk patients. Arch Intern Med 145: 65–69.

Levene DL. (1981) Chest pain: prophet of doom or nagging neurosis? Acta Med Scand 644(suppl): 11–13.

Lopez-Sendon J, Coma-Canella I, Alcasena S et al. (1985) Electrocardiographic findings in acute right ventricular infarction: sensitivity and specificity of electrocardiographic alterations in right precordial leads V4R, V5R, V1, V2, and V3. J Am Coll Cardiol 19: 1273–1279.

Miller DH, Kligfield P, Schreiber TL, Borer JS. (1987) Relationship of prior myocardial infarction to false-positive electrocardiographic diagnosis of acute injury in patients with chest pain. *Arch Intern Med* **147**: 257–261.

Moliterno DJ, Aguirre FV, Cannon CP, Every NP, Granger CB, Sapp SK, Booth JE, Ferguson JJ, for the GUARANTEE Investigators. (1996) The Global Unstable Angina Registry and Treatment Evaluation. *Circulation* **94**: 1.

Morrow DA, Cannon CP, Rifai N *et al.* for the TACTICS-TIMI 18 Investigators. (2001) Ability of minor elevations of troponin I and T to predict benefit from an early invasive strategy in patients with unstable angina and non-ST elevation myocardial infarction: results from a randomized trial. *J Am Med Assoc* **286**: 2405.

Nattel S, Warnica JW, Ogilvie RI. (1980) Indications for admission to a coronary care unit in patients with unstable angina. *Can Med Assoc J* **122**: 180–184.

Nestico PF, Hakki AH, Iskandrian AS *et al.* (1986) Electrocardiographic diagnosis of posterior myocardial infarction revisited. *J Electrocardiol* **19**: 33–40.

Newby LK, Christenson RH, Ohman EM *et al.* (1998) Value of serial troponin T measures for early and late risk stratification in patients with acute coronary syndromes. The GUSTO-IIa Investigators. *Circulation* **98**: 1853.

Pope JH, Ruthazev R, Beshansky JR *et al.* (1998) The clinical presentation of patients with acute cardiac ischaemia in the emergency department: a multicenter controlled clinical trial. *J Thromb Thrombolysis* **6**: 63–74.

Rude RE, Poole WK, Muller JE *et al.* (1983) Electrocardiographic and clinical criteria for recognition of acute myocardial infarction based on analysis of 3,697 patients. *Am J Cardiol* **52**: 936–942.

Sawe U. (1972) Early diagnosis of acute myocardial infarction with special reference to the diagnosis of the intermediate coronary syndrome: a clinical study. *Acta Med Scand* **520**(suppl): 1–76.

Selker HP, Beshansky JR, Griffith JL *et al.* (1998) The use of the ACI-TIPI to assist emergency department triage of patients with chest pain of other symptoms suggestive of acute cardiac ischemia: a multicenter controlled clinical trial. *Ann Intern Med* **129**: 845–55.

Uretsky BF, Farquhar DS, Berezin AF, Hood WB Jr. (1977) Symptomatic myocardial infarction without chest pain: prevalence and clinical course. *Am J Cardiol* **40**: 498–503.

Wrenn KD. (1987) Protocols in the emergency room evaluation of chest pain: do they fail to diagnose lateral wall myocardial infarction? *J Gen Intern Med* **2**: 66–67.

Chapter 5

Initial management

Brian Clapp

> ### Key points
> - As an acute coronary syndrome is a thrombotic process all patients are immediately treated with anti-platelet agents.
> - Patients are monitored in a high-dependency environment and given adequate analgesia and oxygen.
> - In the setting of complete vessel occlusion (ST-elevation) urgent restoration of flow is achieved with thrombolytics or angioplasty.
> - If complete vessel occlusion has not occurred therapy is directed to reduce ischaemia and the development of further thrombus.

5.1 Introduction

The initial management of a patient with an acute coronary syndrome involves general measures, including the use of analgesia and oxygen, and then specific treatments to reduce the short-term and long-term effects of the condition. Although there are similarities, the care pathway divides into two dependent on whether acute total vessel closure is suspected.

Detailed guidelines on the management of acute coronary syndromes have been produced by both the American Cardiac Societies (Krumholz et al. 2006) and the European Cardiac Society (Bassand et al. 2007).

This chapter will describe the generic management pathway and then the important steps in the initial further care in both cases of ST-segment elevation and non-ST–segment elevation.

5.2 First steps

The management of patients with a suspected acute coronary syndrome should occur within a high-dependency area and be directed to prompt and effective triage and initial treatment as time is critical to avoid an adverse outcome.

Patients should be monitored haemodynamically and by continuous electrocardiogram to detect rapidly any deterioration in their clinical condition. Secure intravenous access should be sought and the patient supplied with high-flow oxygen, via a facemask, to maintain arterial saturations above 90 per cent.

5.2.1 Analgesia

Pain is very detrimental to the myocardium during acute ischaemia as it leads to increased oxygen demand by the development of a tachycardia and hypertension. This then causes further ischaemia and potentially increases the degree of cardiac injury and the risk of malignant arrhythmias. Therefore adequate analgesia needs to be administered urgently. While obtaining other routes of delivery, sublingual glyceryl trinitrate (GTN) (2 puffs, 400 mcg) should be given and repeated if required. Unless this relieves all pain this should be supplemented with intravenous opiates (5–10 mg morphine sulphate with an appropriate anti-emetic). Maintenance of adequate arterial oxygen saturations with supplemental oxygen is also important for analgesia in the acute setting.

5.2.2 Anti-platelet agents

As the pathophysiology of acute coronary syndromes involves the development of platelet-rich thrombus within the coronary vessels it is critical to inhibit this process. Multiple pathways in platelet aggregation can be blocked, up to and including the 'final common pathway' of glycoprotein IIb/IIIa receptor binding. In all cases management should include agents to block the cyclo-oxygenase system (aspirin) and the ADP-receptor–dependent pathway (clopidogrel or ticlopidine). The only exception to this is individuals with active and uncontrollable bleeding, for instance intra-cerebrally, or known hypersensitivity. In the acute setting aspirin has an additive effect over thrombolysis and should be initiated at 300 mg (ISIS Group 1988). A loading dose of clopidogrel has also been shown to reduce the composite endpoint of death, myocardial infarction, and stroke from 11.47 per cent to 9.28 per cent (P <0.005) (Fox et al. 2004, Sabatine et al. 2005) and at present the licensed regimen is 300 mg (followed by 75 mg daily). Ex vivo studies have suggested a more rapid time of onset when higher doses are employed and many units have increased this loading dose to 600 mg.

The initial therapeutic strategy is demonstrated in Figure 5.1.

In addition to these general measures specific strategies need to be applied in patients presenting with complications of their acute coronary syndrome (see Chapter 7).

At the end of Figure 5.1 the treatment options can be seen to diverge dependent on whether there is likely to be a completely occluded epicardial vessel (ST-segment elevation) or partially occluded vessel (non-ST–segment elevation). The next sections describe these pathways.

Figure 5.1 Initial therapeutic strategy

Admit patient to high-dependency area

Continuous electrocardiography

High-flow oxygen via face mask

Sublingual glyceryl trinitrate (GTN) (400 mcg; 2 puffs)

Intravenous access

Morphine sulphate 5–10 mg + metoclopramide 10 mg IV

Aspirin 300 mg and clopidogrel 300–600 mg orally

12-lead electrocardiogram

ST-segment elevation   Non-ST–segment elevation

5.3 Management of ST-segment elevation myocardial infarction

Where complete occlusion of the coronary artery has occurred rapid resolution of normal blood flow is required in order to prevent irreversible cell injury. This scenario is diagnosed from the presence of typical chest pain lasting over 20 minutes with significant ST-elevation or new left bundle branch block on the electrocardiogram. Reperfusion can be achieved in three different ways: pharmacologically, by percutaneous coronary intervention or by cardiac surgery. Not all options are available in every setting and the choice of strategy will largely depend upon this.

5.3.1 Thrombolysis

As the vessel is occluded with thrombus agents that act to break down this material are a logical therapeutic approach. A number of different agents have been studied and developed to lyse clots within arteries during a myocardial infarction and the major agents are summarized in Table 5.1.

Hospitals vary on whether they give streptokinase (1.5 mU in 100 mL normal saline infused over 60 minutes) to most patients, reserving tPA or tenecteplase (0.5 mg/kg, 50 mg max) as IV bolus over 10 seconds followed by dalteparin (3000 U IV bolus) for young patients (less than 65 years) with anterior infarcts, or give the latter agent to all comers.

Table 5.1 Major trials of thrombolytic agents			
Agent	**Trial and reference**	**Population**	**Outcome**
Streptokinase	GISSI Lancet 1986; 1: 397–401	11,712 patients with ST-elevation of less than 12 hours duration	21-day mortality reduced from 13% to 10.7% ($P = 0.0002$)
	ISIS-2 ISIS-2 Group 1988	17,187 patients with suspected MI in last 24 hours	Five-week mortality improved 12% to 9.2% ($P < 0.05$) and better if combined with aspirin
Tissue plasminogen activator	ASSET Lancet 1988 II: 525–30	5009 patients with acute myocardial infarction	One-month mortality reduced from 9.8% to 7.2% ($P < 0.05$)
	GISSI-2 Lancet 1990; 336; 65–71	12,381 patients comparing t-PA to streptokinase	No significant difference between the two agents
	TIMI-1 Chesebro et al. 1987	290 patients comparing streptokinase, t-PA, and placebo	No difference in mortality but earlier normalization of flow with t-PA
Tenecteplase	ASSENT-2 Lancet 1999; 354; 716–722	16,949 patients comparing alteplase with tenecteplase	Tenecteplase was as safe and effective as alteplase and easier to administer

Speed of administration is critical. The most benefit is achieved with administration of a thrombolytic within 3 hours of the onset of pain (Widimsky et al. 2003). In some regions thrombolysis is given within the ambulance in order to accelerate the process (Weaver et al. 1990). As speed is important, this is measured and audited as the door-to-needle (or pain-to-needle) time and should ideally be less than 30 minutes. The objective of reperfusion is to achieve normal flow within the epicardial vessel, which from the Thrombolysis in Myocardial Infarction (TIMI) trials has been designated TIMI 3 flow (see definitions in Table 5.2). This, or TIMI 2 flow, is achieved in 62 per cent of patients treated with tissue plasminogen activator and 31 per cent with streptokinase at 90 minutes after administration (Chesebro et al. 1987). Efficacy can also be monitored by the effects of the agents on ST-segment elevation, which is partially correlated with restoration of flow to the epicardial vessel.

Any agent that acts by breaking down clots runs the risk of causing inadvertent bleeding in other territories (Table 5.3). For this reason caution has to be applied in certain settings to balance the risks of the thrombolytic causing unwanted bleeding and the benefits of restoring flow. Debate exists as to which of these contra-indications are absolute or relative and in each individual patient the risk of allowing the infarct to continue has to be balanced against the hazard. If thrombolysis is not possible urgent transfer to a centre able to perform percutaneous coronary intervention needs to be considered, though even in this case the risks of bleeding are still increased.

Table 5.2 TIMI grading

TIMI grade	Definition
Grade 0	No flow
Grade 1	Partial filling of epicardial vessel
Grade 2	Complete, though slow filling
Grade 3	Normal flow within epicardial vessel

Table 5.3 Contraindications to thrombolysis

Absolute contraindications	Relative contraindications
• Major surgery within 1 month	• Hypertension >180/110 mmHg
• Previous haemorrhagic stroke	• Diabetic retinopathy
• Any stroke within last 6 months	• Prolonged cardiopulmonary resuscitation
• Active peptic ulceration or internal bleeding	• Pregnancy
• Possible aortic dissection	• Uncontrolled anticoagulation or bleeding diathesis
• Known intracranial tumour	• Previous streptokinase

Thrombolytics should be administered with careful cardiac and haemodynamic monitoring as they can lead to reperfusion arrhythmias (atrial and ventricular), hypotension, and allergic reactions (in the case of streptokinase). Profound hypotension or allergy will require slowing or stopping of the agent, though it should be continued with arrhythmias and these managed as detailed in later chapters.

5.3.2 Percutaneous coronary intervention

In an appropriately staffed and equipped unit the restoration of normal blood flow (TIMI 3) in the epicardial vessel can be achieved more effectively with percutaneous coronary intervention (PCI). After visualizing the coronary anatomy the occluded or target vessel is crossed with a fine guidewire and a balloon is inflated to restore flow. Usually the procedure will also require the insertion of a coronary stent to optimize the final result. The speed of restoration of flow is paramount and is measured as the door-to-balloon time.

Multiple studies have compared the efficacy of thrombolytics to percutaneous coronary intervention, culminating in a meta-analysis showing the superiority of primary PCI (Keeley *et al.* 2003). Outcome is strongly dependent on the quality of the team and speed of action of the unit involved and favours the development of high-volume specialist centres. Various studies have looked at off-setting the advantages of PCI as a primary strategy against the delay in reperfusion that transferring patients entails (Widimsky *et al.* 2003). In a well-organized system where delays are kept to less than three hours this option offers a better long-term outcome (Anderson *et al.* 2003).

Table 5.4 Comparison of primary angioplasty with fibrinolysis for acute myocardial infarction

Outcome	Primary angioplasty	Fibrinolysis	Odds ratio
• Death	7%	9%	0.73 (0.62–0.86)
• Reinfarction	3%	7%	0.35 (0.27–0.45)
• Stroke	1%	2%	0.46 (0.30–0.72)
• 30-day mortality	9%	13%	$P < 0.005$
From Keeley *et al.* 2003			

In addition to the mechanical opening of the vessel, studies have shown that aggressive platelet inhibition with glycoprotein IIb/IIIa inhibitors reduces the composite of death, myocardial infarction, and urgent revascularization at 30 days (6 per cent vs 14.6 per cent, $P = 0.01$) and six months (Montalescot *et al.* 2001). Local protocols vary, though the most common regimen is the initiation of abciximab (0.25 mg/kg bolus and 0.125 mcg/kg/min infusion for 12 hours) at the time of presentation prior to intervention. This treatment, particularly as it is combined with heparin, leads to an increased bleeding risk and the contra-indications listed for thrombolysis generally apply.

In the setting of a large thrombus burden within the blood vessel some operators favour the use of thrombus extraction devices or mechanisms to avoid distal embolization. Unfortunately there are no large trials to support these options and the details of their advantages and disadvantages are beyond the scope of this text.

In hypotensive patients, particularly in the context of cardiogenic shock, intervention and long-term outcome can be improved by the use of an intra-aortic balloon pump (Sanborn *et al.* 2000). This is inserted in the catheter laboratory via the femoral artery in individuals without significant peripheral vascular disease. It improves coronary perfusion and reduces cardiac afterload, though it requires continued heparinization and has increased vascular complications.

Due to the practical difficulties in organizing 24-hour primary PCI services a large number of studies have looked at the role of facilitated PCI (where agents are given prior to a definite PCI) and rescue PCI (where PCI is used when thrombolysis has failed). With the exception of abciximab immediately prior to intervention, no trial studying facilitated strategies has been shown to be beneficial, largely due to increased bleeding complications, and this cannot be recommended. Rescue PCI is beneficial when pain and ST-elevation persist 90 minutes after thrombolysis (composite of death, myocardial infarction, stroke, and heart failure reduced from 31 per cent to 15 per cent compared to conservative therapy, *P* < 0.01), though the results are less favourable to primary PCI (Gershlick *et al.* 2005).

5.3.3 **Coronary artery bypass grafting**

Although coronary artery bypass surgery is an effective treatment to restore coronary flow, it is rarely used due to the high operative mortality in patients undergoing operations immediately or within the first seven days of an infarct. It may have a role in cardiogenic shock, though with the increase in the options available percutaneously this is very rarely chosen.

5.4 **Management of non-ST–segment elevation acute coronary syndromes**

The treatment of non-ST elevation acute coronary syndromes involves the commencement of therapy to further reduce platelet aggregation, prevent ischaemia, and risk-stratify the patient. This section describes the commonly used strategies. The use of other agents to improve longer-term prognosis, such as statins and angiotensin-converting enzyme inhibitors, are covered in later chapters.

5.4.1 **Heparin and anti-platelets**

In addition to the oral anti-platelets aspirin and clopidogrel, the coagulation pathways should be inhibited with heparin. Due to improved bioavailability, subcutaneous low molecular weight heparins are preferred over unfractionated preparations (Antman *et al.* 1999). Table 5.5 details the evidence and dosing regimens for these heparins.

Heparin should be continued for 48–72 hours or until after coronary angiography and definitive therapy. At the time of coronary intervention some operators continue to use these heparins, though most supplement them with unfractionated preparations. In patients with renal failure (glomerular filtration rate <30 mL/min) unfractionated heparin should be used.

In high-risk individuals with ongoing chest pain, dynamic electrocardiographic changes, and a raised troponin level, further platelet inhibition is required. The use of eptifibatide (small molecular glycoprotein IIb/IIIa inhibitor) has been shown to reduce the composite endpoint of death and non-fatal myocardial infarcts (7.6 per cent vs 9.1 per cent, $P = 0.01$; PURSUIT Trial Investigators 1998). Due to the increased haemorrhagic complications associated with these agents they should be reserved for high-risk individuals and used as a bridge to coronary angiography and intervention.

5.4.2 **Beta-blockade**

In order to reduce myocardial injury and relieve pain it is important to reduce the ischaemic burden. This is partially achieved by pain relief, though also markedly improved by the early initiation of

Table 5.5 Low molecular weight heparins			
Agent	Trial and reference	Outcome	Dose
Enoxaparin	ESSENCE N Engl J Med 1997, 337; 447–452	Death/infarct/ angina reduced at 14 days (16.6% vs 19.8% placebo, $P = 0.019$)	1 mg/kg twice daily for 2–8 days
	TIMI-11B Antman *et al.* 1999	Death/infarct/ revascularization reduced at 8 days compared to unfractionated heparin (12.4% vs 14.5%, $P = 0.048$)	1 mg/kg twice daily
Dalteparin	FRISC Lancet 1996, 347; 561–568	6-day mortality reduced from 4.8% (placebo) to 1.8%	120 U/kg twice daily for 6 days

beta-blockade. Due to the potential for cardiac destabilization this is usually commenced with a short-acting agent, such as metoprolol (12.5 to 25 mg). In patients with late presentations of full-thickness myocardial infarcts beta-blockers have been shown to improve survival, thought to be mostly by reducing the chance of cardiac rupture (ISIS Group 1986). After initiation the dose can be increased, and then a longer-acting agent substituted. Only in individuals with clear reversible airways disease, rather than fixed chronic obstruction, should rate-slowing calcium channel blockers be used, and even in these cases a cardioselective beta-blocker, such as bisoprolol (2.5–10 mg), can often be tolerated.

5.4.3 **Nitrates**

Although nitrates do not improve survival they can be very effective as analgesia, by opening vessels suffering from the spasm that often accompanies an unstable plaque. Although initially given sublingually they are then usually administered intravenously as an infusion at 1–10 mcg/min. Due to their mechanism of action their effectiveness diminishes with time and if pain is relieved they should be stopped in order to avoid tolerance.

5.4.4 **Revascularization**

Early invasive investigation and subsequent revascularization has been shown to be beneficial (six-month death/myocardial infarction reduced from 12.1 per cent to 9.4 per cent, $P = 0.03$; FRISC II 1999). This ideally should occur within 48 hours, though in many cases this is not practical. Ongoing pain or high-risk features, such as hypotension or dynamic electrocardiographic changes, would favour immediate transfer to a unit able to perform these procedures. The subsequent management of patients who are not urgently transferred for coronary angiography is considered in later chapters.

45

Key references

Anderson HR, Nielsen TT, Rasmussen K, et al. (2003) A comparison of coronary angioplasty with fibrinolytic therapy in acute myocardial infarction. New Engl J Med **349**(8): 733–742.

Antman EM, McCabe CH, Gurfinkel EP, et al. (1999) Thrombolysis in Myocardial Infarction-11B. Circulation **100**: 1593–1601.

Bassand J-P, Hamm CW, Ardissino D, et al. (2007) Guidelines for the diagnosis and treatment of non-ST-segment elevation acute coronary syndromes. Eur Heart J **28**: 1598–1660.

Chesebro JH, Knatterud G, Roberts R, et al. (1987) Thrombolysis in Myocardial Infarction (TIMI) Trial, Phase I: A comparison between intravenous tissue plasminogen activator and intravenous streptokinase. Clinical findings through hospital discharge. Circulation **76**(1):142–54.

Cohen M, Demers C, Gurfinkel EP, et al. (1997) A Comparison of Low-Molecular-Weight Heparin with Unfractionated Heparin for Unstable Coronary Artery Disease. The Efficacy and Safety of Subcutaneous Enoxaparin in Non–Q-Wave Coronary Events Study Group, New Engl J Med 337: 447–52.

Fox KA, Peters RJG, Mehta SR, et al. (2004) Benefits and risks of the combination of clopidogrel and aspirin in patients undergoing surgical revascularization for non-ST-elevation acute coronary syndrome: the Clopidogrel in Unstable angina to prevent Recurrent ischemic Events (CURE) Trial. Circulation 108(14): 1682–1687.

FRISC. (1996) Low-molecular-weight heparin during instability in coronary artery disease, Fragmin during Instability in Coronary Artery Disease (FRISC) study group. Lancet 347(9001): 561–8.

FRISC II. (1999) Fragmin and fast revascularisation during instability in coronary artery disease II. Lancet 354: 701–707.

Gershlick, Stephens-Lloyd A, Hughes S, et al. (2005) Rescue angioplasty after failed thrombolytic therapy for acute myocardial infarction. New Engl J Med 353: 2758–2768.

GISSI. (1986) Effectiveness of intravenous thrombolytic treatment in acute myocardial infarction. Gruppo Italiano per lo Studio della Streptochinasi nell'Infarto Miocardico (GISSI). Lancet 1: 397–401.

GISSI-2. (1990) A factorial randomised trial of alteplase versus streptokinase and heparin versus no heparin among 12,490 patients with acute myocardial infarction. Gruppo Italiano per lo Studio della Sopravvivenza nell'Infarto Miocardico. Lancet 336: 65–71.

ISIS Group. (1986) Randomized trial of intravenous atenolol among 16027 case of suspected acute myocardial infarction. Lancet 304: 57–66.

ISIS Group. (1988) Randomized trial of intravenous streptokinase, oral aspirin, both or neither among 17187 cases of suspected acute myocardial infarction. Lancet 2: 349–360.

Keeley EC, Boura JA, Grines CL, et al. (2003) Primary angioplasty versus intravenous thrombolytic therapy for acute myocardial infarction: a quantitative review of 23 randomised trials. Lancet 361: 13–20.

Krumholz HN, Jeffrey L, Anderson JL, et al. (2006) ACC/AHA clinical performance measures for adults with ST-elevation and non-ST-elevation myocardial infarction: a report of the American College of Cardiology/ American Heart Association Task Force on Performance Measures. Circulation 113(5): 732–761.

Montalescot G, Barragan P, Wittenberg O, et al. (2001) Platelet glycoprotein IIb/IIIa inhibition with coronary stenting for acute myocardial infarction. New Engl J Med 344(25): 1895–1903.

PURSUIT Trial Investigators. (1998) Inhibition of the platelet glycoprotein IIb/IIIa receptor with eptifibatide in patients with acute coronary syndromes. New Engl J Med 339: 436–443.

Sabatine MS, Cannon CP, Gibson CM, et al. (2005) Effect of clopidogrel pretreatment before percutaneous coronary intervention in patients with ST-elevation myocardial infarction treated with fibrinolytics: the PCI-CLARITY study. J Am Med Assoc 294(10): 1224–1232.

Sanborn TA, Sleeper LA, Bates ER, *et al.* (2000) Impact of thrombolysis, intra-aortic balloon pump counterpulsation, and their combination in cardiogenic shock complicating acute myocardial infarction: a report from the SHOCK Trial Registry. *J Am Coll Cardiol* **36**: 1123–1129.

Van De Werf F, Adgey J, Ardissino D, *et al.* (1999) Single-bolus tenecteplase compared with front-loaded alteplase in acute myocardial infarction: the ASSENT-2 double-blind randomised trial. Assessment of the Safety and Efficacy of a New Thrombolytic (ASSENT-2). *Lancet* **354**: 716–22.

Widimsky P, Budesínský T, Vorác D, *et al.* (2003) Long distance transport for PCI versus immediate fibrinolysis in acute myocardial infarction (Prague-2). *Eur Heart J* **24**: 94–104.

Wilcox RG, von der Lippe G, Olsson CG, *et al.* (1988) Trial of tissue plasminogen activator for mortality reduction in acute myocardial infarction. Anglo-Scandinavian Study of Early Thrombolysis. (ASSET). *Lancet* **2**: 525–30.

Weaver WD, Eisenberg MS, Martin JS, *et al.* (1990) Myocardial Infarction Triage and Intervention-1. *J Am Coll Cardiol* **15**: 925–931.

Chapter 6

Subsequent management

Samir Srivastava, Gregory YH Lip

Key points

- Acute coronary syndrome patients have a high risk of recurrence of an ischaemic event.
- Appropriate secondary prevention measures should be taken.
- Aggressive risk factor management and pharmacotherapy can reduce the need for further percutaneous coronary interventional procedures.
- Dual anti-platelet therapy is usually continued for up to 12 months (unless being considered for coronary artery bypass grafting); one agent remains life-long.
- ACE inhibitors have an anti-atherogenic effect and should be used in patients with established atherosclerotic disease.
- Blood pressure should ideally be less than 140/90 mmHg (130/80 in diabetics).
- It is essential to address all lifestyle issues.
- Subsequent PCI can be useful for alleviating cardiac ischaemic symptoms, but does not confer a mortality benefit and is not a superior strategy compared with medical therapy.

6.1 Introduction

Following the initial management phase, patients who present with an acute coronary syndrome (ACS) carry a high risk of recurrence of ischaemic events. This is compounded by the fact that appropriate secondary prevention measures such as lifestyle modification and drug therapies tend to be underused. Therefore the long-term outcome for the patient critically depends on the physician utilizing the multi-disciplinary team for lifestyle counselling, as well as prescribing the necessary pharmacological treatment.

The physician must tailor their management decisions according to the individual patient. Initial treatment strategies include pharmacological therapy as well as coronary revascularization. This chapter addresses these issues and focuses on essential secondary preventative measures, on the basis that aggressive risk factor management improves survival, reduces recurrent ischaemic events and the need for interventional procedures, and improves quality of life (Smith *et al.* 2001).

6.2 Anti-platelet agents

A thrombotic event caused by a ruptured atherosclerotic plaque is the usual underlying mechanism of ACS, and a key pathophysiological role in ACS is platelet activation. Acetylsalicylic acid (aspirin) and thienopyridines (clopidogrel) are necessary both for the acute event and subsequent maintenance therapy following an ACS presentation. Newer P2Y12 inhibitors (e.g. prasugrel) with a more rapid onset of action and more potent receptor affinity are currently being studied in randomized controlled trials.

6.2.1 Aspirin

In the context of ACS, an immediate anti-thrombotic effect is required and this can be achieved by administering a loading dose of aspirin 160–320 mg, which is deemed sufficient to produce rapid and complete inhibition of cyclooxygenase-1 (COX-1) in platelets, thereby limiting the formation of thromboxane A2 and inhibiting platelet aggregation. Higher doses of aspirin are no more effective and adverse effects such as gastrotoxicity become problematic (Patrono 1989).

Within a few days of beginning aspirin at a dose of 75 mg once daily, cyclooxygenase is nearly completely inhibited in platelets, and the available evidence supports daily doses of aspirin administered orally in the range 75–150 mg for the long-term prevention of significant vascular events in patients who are thought to be high-risk (Heart Protection Study Collaborative Group [HPSCG] 2002). Side effects tend to be related to gastrointestinal (GI) intolerance, and the risk of GI bleeding tended to be lowest with doses up to 100 mg daily (Yusuf *et al.* 2001). The use of intravenous aspirin has not been studied in large randomized controlled trials, but it is available as an alternative mode of administration.

6.2.2 Clopidogrel

In addition to aspirin, blocking the adenosine diphosphate (ADP) receptor pathway with clopidogrel leads to further benefit in the form of reduced risk of myocardial infarction and recurrent ischaemia in patients with ACS, with a trend toward lower rates of stroke and death from cardiovascular causes (Yusuf *et al.* 2001). Clopidogrel specifically inhibits the P2Y12 ADP receptor, and consequently blocks platelet aggregation.

Following percutaneous coronary intervention (PCI), clopidogrel and aspirin together are the regimen of choice to prevent stent thrombosis (Gurbel et al. 1999) and guidelines suggest some benefit in continuing both for up to 12 months (Bassand et al. 2007). However, a non-significant increase in life-threatening and fatal bleeding has been observed (Peters et al. 2003), but the Clopidogrel in Unstable angina to prevent Recurrent Events (CURE) trial demonstrated 21 fewer cardiovascular deaths for every 1000 patients treated with clopidogrel, and therefore the overall benefit outweighs the risk.

With regards to limitations, inter-individual variability in response to clopidogrel poses a problem because acute and subacute stent thrombosis remain significant clinical concerns despite therapy with thienopyridines and aspirin, and the patient's clinical outcome may be adversely affected as a result (Steinhubl et al. 2001).

6.3 Angiotensin-converting enzyme (ACE) inhibitors

Patients at high risk for coronary events benefit from ACE inhibitor therapy, with data available from ramipril and perindopril (Fox 2003). Impaired left ventricular (LV) systolic function increases mortality, and ACE inhibitors reduce remodeling and improve survival in this situation. It was initially thought that only patients with heart failure would benefit from ACE inhibitors but this therapy appears to be useful in patients with established atherosclerotic disease, independent of LV function.

The reasons for this beneficial effect become clearer by understanding the putative atherosclerotic process. Angiotensin II, which is suppressed by ACE inhibitors, causes endothelial dysfunction by stimulating the expression of pro-inflammatory genes as well as increasing lipid peroxidation and oxyradical formation. The breakdown of bradykinin is reduced by ACE inhibition, and bradykinin is responsible for improving endothelial function by enhancing nitric oxide production and stimulating the synthesis of tissue plasminogen activator, as well as possessing an anti-proliferative effect. Thus, ACE inhibitors appear to counteract the initiation and progression of atherosclerosis by demonstrating a favourable balance between angiotensin II and bradykinin.

Ongoing trials will address whether renin–angiotensin system blockade with angiotensin receptor blockers would provide similar secondary prevention benefits to the ACE inhibitors.

6.4 Beta-blockers

Patients with impaired left ventricular function following ACS, with or without symptoms of heart failure, should be maintained indefinitely on beta-blockers. They can improve cardiac function because of heart rate reduction, therefore prolonging diastolic filling and coronary diastolic perfusion time, as well as decreasing myocardial oxygen demands, improving myocardial energetics, and reducing myocardial oxidative stress (Lopez-Sendo *et al.* 2004, Kukin *et al.* 1999). This therapy also has anti-ischaemic, anti-arrhythmic, and anti-hypertensive properties. Patients should not receive beta-blockers if there is evidence of significant atrioventricular conduction abnormalities, acute LV dysfunction, or a history of asthma.

6.5 **Statins**

The combination of cholesterol pharmacotherapy with dietary intervention has proven beneficial outcome in patients with any form of coronary artery disease (HPSCG 2002). Statins are initiated in the early phase following ACS because they have plaque stabilization and anti-inflammatory properties, as well as a possible beneficial effect on endothelial function. Furthermore, intensive lipid-lowering therapy aimed at reducing low-density lipoprotein (LDL) cholesterol levels below currently recommended levels (target <70 mg/dL–2 mmol/L) can have additional clinical benefit in patients with stable coronary artery disease (Cannon et al. 2004).

6.6 *Calcium channel blockers*

Most of the evidence relating to the use of these calcium channel blockers in ACS is from small randomized controlled trials. For example, some data are available for verapamil post-myocardial infarction where LV function is preserved, whilst for diltiazem, some benefits are seen in non-Q myocardial infarction (Held *et al.* 1989). These drugs are generally good at relieving symptoms (Theroux *et al.* 1985) but there is limited evidence that they reduce mortality and morbidity post-ACS (Held *et al.* 1989). Where there is LV impairment, verapamil and diltiazem can be detrimental due to their negative inotropic effects. The dihydropyridine calcium antagonists (e.g. nifedipine, amlodipine) have generally neutral effects on major adverse cardiac events post-ACS.

There are three sub-classes of calcium channel blockers, and while they all have different pharmacological effects, they all cause similar coronary vasodilatation. Verapamil and diltiazem have the greatest effect on reducing heart rate, while nifedipine and amlodipine produce marked peripheral arterial vasodilatation. In the context of reversible airways disease where it would not be possible to use beta-blockers, rate-limiting calcium channel blockers can be considered as an alternative symptom relief strategy (particularly rate-limiting ones such as diltiazem) provided there are no contra-indications.

6.7 Blood pressure

The blood pressure should be treated to recommended targets, and should ideally be less than 140/90 mmHg in non-diabetic patients. This can be achieved by initiation and maintenance of lifestyle modifications such as increased physical activity, weight control, reduced alcohol and salt intake, and sensible dietary habits (low-fat dairy products, vegetables, fresh fruit), along with the appropriate pharmacotherapy. Patients with diabetes or chronic renal dysfunction should have a blood pressure of less than 130/80 (De Backer *et al.* 2003).

Given that many patients require combination therapy to achieve blood pressure targets, current guidelines for hypertension management suggest an approach to achieve targets by using the new A/CD algorithm (Figure 6.1), as recommended in the joint National Institute for Health and Clinical Excellence (NICE) and British Hypertension Society (BHS) guidelines (17) (issued on 28 June 2006, available at http://www.nice.org.uk/CG034).

6.8 Diabetes

Patients with diabetes are generally at high risk for adverse events, its presence being an independent predictor of higher mortality among patients with ACS (McGuire *et al.* 2000). There are more comorbid associations such as impaired renal function, heart failure, and stroke (Franklin *et al.* 2004). Every patient presenting with ACS should be investigated for an abnormal fasting blood glucose level. In established diabetics, a combination of pharmacological treatment and lifestyle advice (weight reduction in particular) can be used in an attempt to achieve a HbA1c of 6.5 per cent or less. Blood pressure control is crucial, and the routine use of aspirin, ACE inhibitors, and statins is to be recommended.

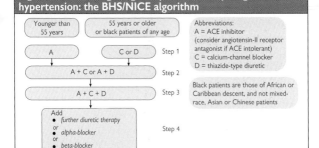

Figure 6.1 Choosing drugs for patients newly diagnosed with hypertension: the BHS/NICE algorithm

6.9 **Lifestyle**

Reducing long-term risk of recurrence of events in ACS patients is not just related to drug therapy. Several lifestyle modifications can also be effective and it is essential that they are addressed. Smoking is a frequent problem; realistically in the long term, many smokers will not abstain, even if they manage to do so after the acute event. Therefore the use of nicotine replacement and counselling should be made available. A healthy diet and regular physical exercise should also be encouraged. Chronic aerobic exercise has been shown to increase high-density lipoprotein (HDL) cholesterol levels (Kelley *et al.* 2006). Low HDL is associated with an increased risk of death from coronary artery disease (Gordon *et al.* 1986).

6.10 **Need for further intervention**

With increased operator experience, new technology, and adjunctive pharmacological therapy, the overall success of percutaneous coronary intervention has improved and the complication rate is less. PCI is now associated with mortality and a need for emergency bypass surgery in less than 1 per cent of cases. However, restenosis requiring a second revascularization procedure remains a limitation. Following PCI, platelets and fibrin adhere to the site within minutes of vessel injury, with subsequent inflammatory cell infiltration and migration of vascular smooth muscle cells towards the lumen. After 6 months, the repair process enhances stability and the risk of restenosis decreases significantly. The success of PCI can be defined by angiographic, procedural, and clinical criteria.

With regards to subsequent PCI in symptomatic patients who are already beyond the acute presentation with ACS, randomized controlled trials have shown that PCI in patients with non-acute coronary disease may result in greater relief from angina than medical treatment, but the magnitude of this effect varies considerably and there is no mortality benefit achieved with intervention over medical therapy (Bucher *et al.* 2000).

If there is an indication for myocardial revascularization in the follow-up period following ACS, the preferred approach (PCI or coronary artery bypass grafting) will depend on the patient's symptoms, comorbidities, and the severity of the coronary lesions as demonstrated on angiography.

Key references

Bassand J-P, Hamm CW, Ardissino D, Boersma E, Budaj A, Fernandez-Aviles F, Fox KAA, Hasdai DE, Ohman M, Wallentin L, Wijns W. (2007) Guidelines for the diagnosis and treatment of non-ST-segment elevation acute coronary syndromes. *Eur Heart J* **28**: 1598–1660.

Bucher HC, Hengstler P, Schindler C, Guyatt GH. (2000) Percutaneous transluminal coronary angioplasty versus medical treatment for non-acute coronary heart disease: meta-analysis of randomised controlled trials. *Br Med J* **321**: 73–77.

Cannon CP, Braunwald E, McCabe CH, Rader DJ, Rouleau JL, Belder R, Joyal SV, Hill KA, Pfeffer MA, Skene AM, for the Pravastatin or Atorvastatin Evaluation and Infection Therapy. Thrombolysis in Myocardial Infarction 22 Investigators. (2004) Comparison of intensive and moderate lipid lowering with statins after acute coronary syndromes. *New Engl J Med* **350**: 1495–1504.

De Backer G, Ambrosioni E, Borch-Johnsen K, Brotons C, Cifkova R, Dallongeville J, Ebrahim S, Faergeman O, Graham I, Mancia G, Manager Cats V, Orth-Gomer K, Perk J, Pyorala K, Rodicio JL, Sans S, Sansoy V, Sechtem U, Silber S, Thomsen T, Wood D. (2003) European guidelines on cardiovascular disease prevention in clinical practice. Third Joint Task Force of European and Other Societies on Cardiovascular Disease Prevention in Clinical Practice. *Eur Heart J* **24**: 1601–1610.

Fox KM. The European Trial on Reduction of Cardiac Events With Perindopril in Stable Coronary Artery Disease (EUROPA) Investigators. (2003) Efficacy of perindopril in reduction of cardiovascular events among patients with stable coronary artery disease: randomised, double-blind, placebo-controlled, multicentre trial (the EUROPA study). *Lancet* **362**(9386). 782–788.

Franklin K, Goldberg RJ, Spencer F, Klein W, Budaj A, Brieger D, Marre M, Steg PG, Gowda N, Gore JM. (2004) Implications of diabetes in patients with acute coronary syndromes. The Global Registry of Acute Coronary Events. *Arch Intern Med* **164**: 1457–1463.

Gordon DJ, Knoke J, Probstfield JL, Superko R, Tyroler HA. (1986) High-density lipoprotein cholesterol and coronary heart disease in hypercholesterolemic men: the Lipid Research Clinic Coronary Primary Prevention Trial. *Circulation* **74**: 1217–1225.

Gurbel PA, O'Connor CM, Cummings CC, Serebruany VL. (1999) Clopidogrel: the future choice for preventing platelet activation during coronary stenting? *Pharm Res* **65**: 109–123.

Heart Protection Study Collaborative Group. (2002) MRC/BHF Heart Protection Study of cholesterol lowering with simvastatin in 20,536 high-risk individuals: a randomized placebo-controlled trial. *Lancet* **360** (9326): 7–22.

Held PH, Yusuf S, Furberg CD. (1989) Calcium channel blockers in acute myocardial infarction and unstable angina: an overview. *Br Med J* **299**: 1187–1192.

Kelley GA, Kelley KS, Franklin B. (2006) Aerobic exercise and lipids and lipoproteins in patients with cardiovascular disease: a meta-analysis of randomized controlled trials. *J Cardiopulm Rehabil* **26**: 131–139.

Kukin ML, Kalman J, Charney RH, Levy DK, Buchholz-Varley C, Ocampo ON, Eng C. (1999) Prospective, randomized comparison of effect of long-term treatment with metoprolol or carvedilol on symptoms, exercise, ejection fraction, and oxidative stress in heart failure. *Circulation* **99**: 2645–2651.

Lopez-Sendo J, Swedberg K, McMurray J, Tamargo J, Maggioni AP, Dargie H, Tendera M, Waagstein F, Kjekshus J. Task Force Members. (2004) Expert consensus document on β-adrenergic receptor blockers: the Task Force on Beta-Blockers of the European Society of Cardiology. *Eur Heart J* **25**(15): 1341–1362.

McGuire DK, Emanuelsson H, Granger CB, Magnus Ohman E, Moliterno DJ, White HD, Ardissino D, Box JW, Califf RM, Topol EJ. GUSTO-IIb Investigators. (2000) Influence of diabetes mellitus on clinical outcomes across the spectrum of acute coronary syndromes. Findings from the GUSTO-IIb study. *Eur Heart J* **21**: 1750–1758.

NICE/BHS. (2006) Hypertension: management of hypertension in adults in primary care. http://www.nice.org.UK/CGO34 (accessed 16/11/07).

Patrono C. (1989) Aspirin and human platelets: from clinical trials to acetylation of cyclooxygenase and back. *Trends Pharmacol Sci* **10**: 453–458.

Peters RJ, Mehta SR, Fox KA, Zhao F, Lewis BS, Kopecky SL, Diaz R, Commerford PJ, Valentin V, Yusuf S. Clopidogrel in Unstable angina to prevent Recurrent Events (CURE) trial investigators. (2003) Effects of aspirin dose when used alone or in combination with clopidogrel in patients with acute coronary syndromes: observations from the Clopidogrel in Unstable angina to prevent Recurrent Events (CURE) study. *Circulation* **108**: 1682–1687.

Smith SC Jr, Dove JT, Jacobs AK, Kennedy JW, Kereiakes D, Kern MJ, Kuntz RE, Popma JJ, Schaff HV, Williams DO, Gibbons RJ, Alpert JP, Eagle KA, Faxon DP, Fuster V, Gardner TJ, Gregoratos G, Russell RO. (2001) ACC/AHA guidelines for percutaneous coronary intervention (revision of the 1993. PTCA guidelines): executive summary. *J Am Coll Cardiol* **37**(8): 2215–2239.

Steinhubl SR, Talley JD, Braden GA, Tcheng JE, Casterella PJ, Moliterno DJ, Navetta FI, Berger PB, Popma JJ, Dangas G, Gallo R, Sane DC, Saucedo JF, Jia G, Lincoff AM, Theroux P, Holmes DR, Teirstein PS, Kereiakes DJ. (2001) Point of care measured platelet inhibition correlates with a reduced risk of an adverse cardiac event after percutaneous coronary intervention: results of the GOLD (AU-Assessing Ultegra) multicenter study. *Circulation* **103**: 2528–2530.

Theroux P, Taeymans Y, Morissette D, Bosch X, Pelletier GB, Waters DD. (1985) A randomized study comparing propranolol and diltiazem in the treatment of unstable angina. *J Am Coll Cardiol* **5**: 717–722.

Yusuf S, Zhao F, Mehta SR, Chrolavicius S, Tognoni G, Fox KK. (2001) Effects of clopidogrel in addition to aspirin in patients with acute coronary syndromes without ST-segment elevation. *New Engl J Med* **345**: 494–502.

Chapter 7

Complications

Ian Webb, Michael Marber

Key points

- A significant proportion of patients presenting with an acute coronary syndrome will suffer complications either as a direct result of myocardial ischaemia or secondary to medical therapy and intervention.
- Complications can occur during the index admission or many years later.
- Major risk factors include increasing age and number of comorbidities, female sex, and the extent of myocardial ischaemia and necrosis.
- Targeted therapy, in-patient monitoring and longer-term surveillance are important in limiting complications and ensuring their prompt detection and appropriate initiation of therapy.

7.1 Introduction

Complications of acute coronary syndromes (ACS) encompass a diverse group of pathologies, which can occur acutely at the time of presentation or much later as a consequence of permanent myocardial damage. Contemporary therapeutic strategies have undoubtedly impacted on this risk, but in doing so have increased the incidence of iatrogenic complications.

7.2 Dysrhythmia

Rhythm disturbances may result from ischaemia or successful reperfusion, or as a chronic feature of a scarred and dilated ventricle. The presence, prognostic implication, and treatment aims are defined by the nature of dysrhythmia, the temporal relation to ACS presentation, and the extent of structural damage to the heart.

7.2.1 **Ventricular dysrhythmia**

7.2.1.1 *Ischaemia and reperfusion*

Ischaemia-driven dysrhythmias are a frequent cause of death in acute myocardial infarction (MI). Primary ventricular fibrillation (VF), defined by the absence of preceding hypotension or heart failure, affects 3–5 per cent of survivors-to-hospital with MI, with a peak occurrence in the first 4 hours. Risk factors identified by a recent meta-analysis (Gheeraert *et al.* 2006) are shown in Box 7.1.

Reperfusion dysrhythmias include ventricular tachycardia (VT), VF, and accelerated idioventricular rhythms. They are common and self-limiting, and generally require no specific intervention. Presence correlates with successful coronary artery recanalization, distal microvascular perfusion, and ST-segment resolution on ECG (Ilia *et al.* 2003). Initial management of all patients with ventricular dysrhythmias should be guided by national advanced life-support protocols. Direct current cardioversion (DCCV) is mandated if the patient is haemodynamically compromised or symptomatic. IV amiodorone is recommended for sustained or recurrent VT, particularly where left ventricular (LV) function is unknown. Lidocaine is a useful anti-dysrhythmic, but its prophylactic use has been associated with increased risk of fatal bradycardia and asystole (Hine *et al.* 1989). Beta-blockers should be administered to all suspected MI patients unless contra-indicated, and hypokalaemia and hypomagnesaemia corrected promptly.

7.2.1.2 *Late ventricular dysrhythmias (ischaemic cardiomyopathy)*

Late ventricular dysrhythmias complicate an impaired and scarred ventricle, and carry an adverse prognosis. Risk assessment involves knowledge of LV function, presence of inducible ischaemia and symptom control. Current UK guidelines recommend implantable cardiac defibrillator (ICD) therapy for primary and secondary prevention according to defined criteria.

Box 7.1 **Risk factors for ventricular dysrhythmia**
Demographics:
• Increasing age
• Male sex
• No prior history of ischaemic heart disease (IHD)
• Smoking history
ACS presentation:
• ST-elevation MI
• Preceding atrioventricular block
• Lowered admission heart rate
• Lowered admission potassium

Routine post-MI care should include beta-blockers, ACE inhibitors, and statin therapy, all of which are associated with reduced VT/VF and risk of sudden cardiac death (SCD). Amiodorone and other anti-dysrhythmic therapy may be required for additional symptom control. VT ablation is reserved for intractable symptoms (NICE Guidelines 2006; see Table 7.1).

7.2.2 Atrial fibrillation

Atrial fibrillation (AF) presents in approximately 15 per cent of ACS patients. Half of these are defined as new-onset during admission (Mehta *et al.* 2003). Identified risk factors from the Global Registry of Acute Coronary Events (GRACE) registry are shown in Box 7.2.

New-onset AF is associated with an adverse in-hospital outcome, including increased risk of shock, left ventricular failure (LVF), cardiac arrest, re-infarction, stroke, and major bleeding complications. Treatment is targeted at rate-control, ideally with beta-blockers in the absence of haemodynamic instability or uncontrolled LVF. Rarely, cardioversion is indicated for sustained or compromising fibrillation.

Table 7.1 NICE guidelines for ICD implantation (2006)	
Primary prevention	**Secondary prevention (in the absence of reversible causes)**
Previous MI (≥4 weeks) and: *either* • LVEF ≤35% (and ≤NYHA III) AND • Non-sustained VT on Holter AND • Inducible VT on EP testing *or* • LVEF ≤30% (and ≤NYHA III) AND • QRS duration ≥120 msec	• Survivors of cardiac arrest due to either VT or VF • Spontaneous sustained VT causing syncope or haemodynamic compromise • Sustained VT without syncope or cardiac arrest , with EF ≤35% (and ≤NYHA III)

Abbreviations: ICD = implantable cardiac defibrillator; MI = myocardial infarction; LVEF = left-ventricular ejection fraction; NYHA = New York Health Association; VT = ventricular tachycardia; EP = electro-physiology; VF = ventricular fibrillation.

Box 7.2 Risk factors for atrial fibrillation

Demographics:
- Increasing age
- Female sex
- Hypertension

ACS presentation:
- Myocardial infarction
- Cardiac arrest
- ≥ Killip class II heart failure
- Raised resting heart rate
- Lowered systolic blood pressure

7.2.3 **Conduction disturbances**

Transient sinus bradycardia and atrioventricular (AV) block are common after inferior myocardial infarction, but only infrequently result in haemodynamic instability requiring intervention. The incidence of high-grade (second- or third-degree) AV block is less now with revascularization, but may still complicate up to 20 per cent of inferior infarcts. Atropine and temporary pacing may be required. Progression to permanent pacing beyond 10–14 days post-MI is rare (<1 per cent). Complete heart block is associated with larger inferior infarcts and a significant increase in in-patient mortality. High-degree AV block with anterior myocardial infarction signifies extensive septal necrosis with high risk of cardiogenic shock and progression to ventricular standstill. Temporary pacing is mandatory in this setting.

7.3 **Ventricular dysfunction**

Primary pump failure (LVF and cardiogenic shock) and anatomical complications of infarction appear to be declining with contemporary revascularization strategies and implementation of aggressive medical therapy (Fox *et al.* 2007). Ischaemic cardiomyopathy, however, remains a leading cause of chronic heart failure with poor long-term prognosis.

7.3.1 **Acute pulmonary oedema**

This complicates up to 40 per cent of ACS admissions and is commonly due to LV systolic dysfunction (Table 7.2). A significant number of patients with clinical signs of heart failure, however, will have preserved systolic function on echocardiography (diastolic dysfunction). Both confer an increase in hospital complications and an adverse longer-term prognosis (Moller *et al.* 2003).

Supportive treatment includes the use of loop diuretics, intravenous nitrates, and opiates in order to achieve respiratory stability through a reduction in preload, afterload, and myocardial oxygen demand.

Table 7.2 **Causes of acute pulmonary oedema and hypotension in ACS patients**	
1. Acute pulmonary oedema	**2. Hypotension with ACS**
• Acute LV dysfunction (diastolic ± systolic)	• Iatrogenic drug-induced
• Mitral valve rupture or ischaemic regurgitation	• LV (or RV) shock
	• VSD or free wall rupture
• Dysrhythmias (tachy- or bradycardia)	• Mitral valve rupture and severe MR
	• Tamponade
• Ventricular septal rupture	• Dysrhythmia
	• Bleeding
Abbreviations: ACS = acute coronary syndromes; LV = left ventricular; RV = right ventricular; VSD = ventricular septal defect; MR = mitral regurgitation	

Continuous positive airway pressure (CPAP) for severe pulmonary oedema reduces progression to mechanical ventilation and improves in-hospital survival (Peter *et al.* 2006).

Other prognostic interventions based on large clinical trial data include eplerenone for manifest pulmonary oedema, ACE inhibitor or angiotensin receptor blocker (ARB) therapy, and beta-blockers once haemodynamically stable and pulmonary oedema controlled (Table 7.3).

Table 7.3 Early therapy for post-MI patients with heart failure (HF)

Trial and drug class	Trial design	Therapy	Relative risk reduction
ACE inhibitors			
SAVE (1994)	n = 2231; 3–16 d post-MI EF <40% Mean follow-up 42 months	Captopril	↓19% mortality ↓25% repeat MI
AIRE (1997)	n = 2006; 3–10 d post-MI Clinical HF Mean follow-up 15 months	Ramipril	↓27% mortality ↓30% SCD
AIREX (1997)	3-y follow-up of 603 UK patients from AIRE study	Ramipril	↓36% mortality
TRACE (1995)	n = 1749; 3–7 d post-MI EF <35% and/or clinical HF 24–50-month follow-up	Trandolapril	↓18% mortality ↓24% SCD ↓29% severe HF
Angiotensin II receptor blockers			
VALIANT (2003)	n = 14,703; 0.5–10 d post-MI EF <35% and/or clinical HF Median follow-up 24.7 months	Captopril, valsartan or both	Comparable between groups ↑ drug intolerance with dual therapy
OPTIMAAL (2002)	n = 5477; <10 d post-MI EF <35% and/or clinical HF Mean follow-up 2.7 years	Losartan or captopril	Trend towards ↑ mortality and morbidity in losartan group
Aldosterone antagonists			
EPHESUS (2003)	n = 6642; 3–14 d post-MI EF <40% and clinical HF Mean follow-up 16 months	Eplerenone	↓15% mortality ↓17%CV death

Table 7.3 (Contd.)			
Trial and drug class	Trial design	Therapy	Relative risk reduction
Beta-blockers			
CAPRICORN (2001)	n = 1959; 3–21 d post-MI EF < 40%. Stable on ACE inhibitors Mean follow-up 1.3 y	Carvedilol	↓20% mortality ↓21% CV death ↓50% non-fatal MI

Abbreviations: SAVE = Survival And Ventricular Enlargement (Rutherford et al. 1994); AIRE = Acute Infarction Ramipril Efficacy (Cleland et al. 1997); AIREX = AIRE Extension (Hall et al. 1997); TRACE = Trandolapril Cardiac Evaluation (Kober et al. 1995); VALIANT = Valsartan In Acute Myocardial Infarction Trial (Pfeffer et al. 2003); OPTIMAAL = Optimal Therapy In Myocardial Infarction with the Angiotensin II Antagonist Losartan (Dickstein et al. 2002); EPHESUS = Eplerenone Postacute Myocardial Infarction Heart Failure Efficacy and Survival Study (Pitt et al. 2003); CAPRICORN = Carvedilol Post Infarct Survival Control in LV Dysfunction (Dargie 2001).

7.3.2 Cardiogenic shock

Cardiogenic shock complicates up to 10 per cent of acute myocardial infarcts and carries a significant mortality, particularly if present by the time of admission to hospital. Shock physiology is seen with a variety of ACS complications (see Table 7.2) for which echocardiography is mandated to differentiate between them. It is defined clinically by a triad of features (Box 7.3).

7.3.2.1 Acute LV shock

Data from the SHOCK registry demonstrate that urgent multi-vessel PCI or coronary artery bypass grafting (CABG) supported by intra-aorta balloon pump (IABP) and inotrope therapy is superior to medical therapy alone and should be undertaken as soon as possible (Hochman et al. 1999). A trend towards better survival for medical therapy in ≥75-year-olds has been suggested, and the merits of invasive strategies beyond 12–24 hours of developing shock physiology remain debatable. Ventricular assist devices and cardiac transplantation form the final option but are rarely available.

7.3.2.2 Acute RV shock

RV infarction complicates 30–40 per cent of inferior MIs, half of which may demonstrate haemodynamic instability. Presentation is with systemic hypotension, elevated right atrial pressure, and clear lung fields, raising the differential of tamponade or massive pulmonary embolus. RV shock, however, should always be suspected in the context of inferoposterior MI and ST-segment elevation in the right precordial leads (especially rV4). Revascularization should be undertaken where appropriate, and patients may require transient inotrope and IABP support. However, haemodynamic stability is often restored simply by appropriate fluid resuscitation in order to elevate RV preload and thereby enhance pulmonary perfusion and LV filling (Kinch et al. 1994).

Box 7.3 Clinical definition of cardiogenic shock

- Sustained arterial hypotension (SBP <90 mmHg for ≥30 mins)
- Pump failure (CI ≤2.2 L/min and PAWP ≥15 mmHg)
- End-organ hypoperfusion (e.g. oliguria ≤30 mL/h)

Abbreviations: SBP = systolic blood pressure; PAWP = pulmonary artery wedge pressure; CI = cardiac index.

Table 7.4 Treatment of LVF complicating ACS

Normotensive or hypertensive patient	Hypotensive patient
• High-flow O_2 (60–100%)	• High-flow O_2 (60–100%)
• IV GTN (10–100 mcg/min)	• Invasive monitoring ± respiratory support
• IV morphine (5–10 mg)	
• IV frusemide 40–100 mg bolus or 5–20 mg/h infusion	• Dobutamine (2.5–10 mcg/kg/min) ± dopamine or epinephrine
• CPAP	• Urgent echo to exclude:
• IABP (if active ischaemia)	VSD/free wall rupture
• ACS protocol including revascularization as appropriate	Acute severe MR (rupture)
	Tamponade
• ACE inhibitor/ARB within 24 h	Acute valve dysfunction
• Eplerenone	• IABP and revascularization (if active ischaemia)
• Beta-blocker	

Abbreviations: ACS = acute coronary syndromes; IV = intravenous; GTN = glyceryl trinitrate; CPAP = continuous positive airway pressure; IABP = intra-aortic balloon pump; ACE = angiotensin-converting enzyme; ARB = angiotensin receptor blocker; VSD = ventricular septal defect; MR = mitral regurgitation.

7.3.2.3 *Ventricular free wall rupture and septal perforation*

Free wall rupture complicates <1 per cent of infarctions but is universally fatal untreated and carries a 30-day mortality of 40 per cent even after surgical repair (SHOCK study). Implicated risk factors from registry data are summarized in Table 7.5. Forty per cent of events will occur within the first 24 hours of infarction and 85 per cent by the end of the first week. Patients present with evolving tamponade physiology, persistent ST-segment elevation in spite of revascularization, and occasionally profound bradycardia progressing to pulseless electrical activity in end-stage cases. Ventricular septal rupture is even less common but carries an 87 per cent mortality at 30 days post-repair and 96 per cent in those managed medically. The majority of patients present with haemodynamic compromise coincident with a new systolic murmur, with or without thrill. Pulmonary oedema results from left ventricular dysfunction (in anterior infarcts) exacerbated by left-to-right shunting of blood.

Echocardiography is mandated where ventricular septal or free wall rupture is suspected. Haemodynamic support with inotropes and IABP therapy may be required pending transfer to a cardiothoracic facility for consideration of revascularization and surgical repair.

Table 7.5 Risk factors for LV free wall and septal rupture

Rupture type	Demographics	ACS presentation
LV free wall ruture	• Increased age • Female sex • No previous history of MI	• Transmural anterior MI • Failure to reperfuse/ TIMI 0 flow at angiography
Ventricular septal rupture	• Increased age • Female sex • Hypertension	• Transmural anterior MI • Killip class III–IV heart failure

7.3.2.4 *Acute mitral regurgitation*

New-onset mitral incompetence post-infarction carries an adverse prognosis due to primary valve dysfunction itself as well as the extent of infarction causing it. Acute papillary muscle rupture, in particular, may present as an acute surgical emergency with florid pulmonary oedema, new systolic murmur of MR, and evolving cardiogenic shock. It typically presents within the first few days after MI, with a 24-hour mortality of 50 per cent untreated (Nishimura *et al.* 2000). Postero-medial papillary muscle rupture with inferoposterior MI is ~10 times more likely than anterolateral papillary involvement, which receives a dual blood supply from both left anterior descending (LAD) and circumflex arteries. Diagnosis is confirmed with echocardiography. Supportive management with intropes, afterload reduction, and IABP therapy may be required as an interim measure pending emergency surgical repair. Simultaneous revascularization and the ability to repair rather than replace the valve are associated with better outcome (Kishon *et al.* 1992).

Table 7.6 Causes of post-MI mitral regurgitation and risk factors associated with acute papillary muscle rupture

Causes of post-MI mitral regurgitation	Risk factors for acute papillary muscle rupture
• Ruptured papillary muscle • Ruptured chordae tendinae • Annular dilatation and functional MR secondary to LV dilatation • Incomplete leaflet closure secondary to regional wall motion abnormality • Worsening of pre-existing MR	• Age • Female sex • Inferoposterior MI • Single-vessel disease • Non-diabetic patients

7.3.3 Chronic ischaemic cardiomyopathy

Ischaemic heart disease has been identified as a leading cause of chronic heart failure in multiple population-based studies and large therapeutic trials. Mortality remains high in spite of advances in therapy with contemporary 5-year survival rates of 35–59 per cent (Levy et al. 2002, Bleumink et al. 2004, Roger et al. 2004). Management is beyond the scope of this chapter, but should include medical therapy with beta-blockers, ACE inhibitors, and diuretics. ARBs, digoxin, aldosterone antagonists, and hydralazine/nitrate therapy are reserved for certain patient sub-groups. Revascularization may be considered where there is evidence of reversible ischaemia. Cardiac resynchronization therapy with biventricular pacing and implantable cardiac defibrillators are indicated for advanced symptomatic disease according to defined criteria (American College of Cardiology (ACC)/American Heart Association (AHA) guidelines; Hunt et al. 2005).

7.3.4 LV aneurysm formation

LV aneurysms of varying size may develop in up to 15 per cent of transmural infarct survivors, and are typically associated with LAD infarcts and failure to achieve reperfusion. Over 75 per cent are therefore located to the anteroapical position, and clinical suspicion should be raised in the presence of late post-MI ventricular dysrhythmias, persistent ST-segment elevation on ECG, and in patients with systemic emboli soon after infarction. Diagnosis and viability can be confirmed by a variety of modalities including stress echocardiography and perfusion-magnetic resonance imaging. Treatment is directed at rhythm control, management of heart failure, and prophylactic anti-coagulation. Surgical repair is advocated only for refractory symptoms.

7.4 Pericardial effusions and inflammatory complications

Three major pericardial-related complications can arise in ACS patients. The prevalence of each increases with size of infarct sustained and, accordingly, is associated with increased morbidity and mortality. The overall incidence, however, appears to be declining with contemporary revascularization strategies.

7.4.1 Infarction pericarditis

This will affect 5–20 per cent of patients and usually occurs within the first 3 days post-MI. There is a higher relative risk in anterior transmural infarcts. Patients may complain of pericarditic pain and a precordial rub may be audible. ECG changes are often masked by those of the antecedent infarct, but atypical T-wave progression or 'normalization' of T-wave inversion strongly support the diagnosis.

Transient atrial fibrillation may also present at this time. Echocardiography is recommended to exclude significant effusions, for which heparin anti-coagulation should be discontinued in the absence of ongoing ischaemia. Other than aspirin, non-steroidal anti-inflammatory drugs (NSAIDs) and steroids should be avoided due to the detrimental effect on infarct healing and coronary blood flow. Treatment with paracetamol and opioid analgesia is usually effective.

7.4.2 **Pericardial effusion**

The time course and risk factors for developing pericardial effusions mirror those of infarction pericarditis. Up to 28 per cent of ACS patients in prospective studies demonstrate reactive pericardial effusions, peaking at 3 days post-MI and with a higher relative risk in transmural anterior infarcts and associated pulmonary oedema (Galve et al. 1986). This group intrinsically carries an adverse prognosis, but the presence of pericardial effusion itself only rarely causes tamponade physiology requiring emergency drainage. The presence of echodense thrombus within the pericardial space on echocardiography increases the sensitivity and specificity for detecting cardiac rupture. This is associated with a heavy blood-stained pericardial aspirate, and emergency surgical repair should be considered.

7.4.3 **Dressler's syndrome**

This is considered a reactive autoimmune response to infarction (or cardiac surgery), defined clinically by fever, pleuro-pericarditis, and raised inflammatory markers (C-reactive protein (CRP) and erythrocyte sedimentation rate (ESR)). It typically presents weeks to months after infarction, but occasionally will manifest as a continuation of infarction pericarditis. Incidence in the reperfusion era is <0.5 per cent and it tends to run a benign course. Echocardiography will exclude significant effusions and pericardiocentesis is again rarely necessary. Treatment should include NSAID therapy (if a reasonable time has elapsed post-MI) and corticosteroids may help with protracted symptoms.

7.5 **Iatrogenic complications**

Increasingly, aggressive therapy for ACS patients and an ageing population predispose to a myriad of potential iatrogenic complications. A comprehensive list is beyond the scope of this chapter, but it is worth noting that the major ACS clinical trials have a 2–40 per cent risk of major adverse complications and patient drop-out. ACE inhibitors, beta-blockers, and statins all demonstrate adverse pharmacological profiles, but arguably the most significant iatrogenic complication relates to haemorrhagic risk with thrombolysis, anti-platelet agents, and anti-coagulation.

Key references

Bleumink GS, Knetsch AM, Sturkenboom MC, et al. (2004) Quantifying the heart failure epidemic: prevalence, incidence rate, lifetime risk and prognosis of heart failure. The Rotterdam Study. *Eur Heart J* **25**(18): 1614–1619.

Cleland JG, Erhardt L, Murray G, et al. (1997) Effect of ramipril on morbidity and mode of death among survivors of acute myocardial infarction with clinical evidence of heart failure. A report from the AIRE Study Investigators. *Eur Heart J* **18**(1): 41–51.

Dargie HJ. (2001) Effect of carvedilol on outcome after myocardial infarction in patients with left ventricular dysfunction: the CAPRICORN randomized trial. *Lancet* **357**: 1385–1390.

Dickstein K, Kiekhus J, et al. (2002) Effects of losartan and captopril on mortality and morbidity in high-risk patients after acute myocardial infarction: the OPTIMAAL randomized trial. Optimal Trial in Myocardial Infarction with Angiotensin II Antagonist Losartan. *Lancet* **360**: 752–760.

Fox KA, Steg PG, Eagle KA, et al. (2007) Decline in rates of death and heart failure in acute coronary syndromes, 1999–2006. *J Am Med Assoc* **297**(17): 1892–1900.

Galve E, Garcia-del-Castillo H, Evangelista A, et al. (1986) Pericardial effusion in the course of myocardial infarction: incidence, natural history, and clinical relevance. *Circulation*; **73**(2): 294–9.

Gheeraert PJ, De Buyzere ML, Taeymans YM, et al. (2006) Risk factors for primary ventricular fibrillation during acute myocardial infarction: a systematic review and meta-analysis. *Eur Heart J* **27**: 2499–510.

Hall AS, Murray GD, and Ball SG. (1997) Follow-up of patients randomly allocated ramipril or placebo for heart failure after acute myocardial infarction: AIRE Extension (AIREX) Study. *Lancet* **349**: 1493–1497.

Hine LK, Laird N, Hewitt P, and Chalmers TC. (1989) Meta-analytical evidence against prophylactic use of lidocaine in acute myocardial infarction. *Arch Intern Med* **149**(12): 2694–2698.

Hochman JS, Sleeper LA, Webb JG, et al. (1999) Early revascularisation in acute myocardial infarction complicated by cardiogenic shock. *New Engl J Med* **341**: 625–634.

Hunt SA. (2005) ACC/AHA 2005 Guideline update for the diagnosis and management of chronic heart failure in the adult. *J Am Coll Cardiol* **46**: 1116–1143.

Ilia R, Amit G, Cafric, et al. (2003) Reperfusion arrhythmias during coronary angiography for acute myocardial infarction predict ST-segment resolution. *Coron Artery Dis* **14**(6): 439–441.

Kinch J, and Ryan TJ. (1994) Right ventricular infarction. *New Engl J Med* **17**: 1211–1217.

Kishon Y, Oh JK, Schaff HV, et al. (1992) Mitral valve operation in post infarction rupture of a papillary muscle: immediate results and long-term follow-up in 22 patients. *Mayo Clin Proc* **67**: 1023–1030.

Køber L, Torp-Pederson C, Carlson JE, et al. (1995) A clinical trial of the angiotensin-converting-enzyme inhibitor trandolapril in patients with left ventricular dysfunction after myocardial infarction. Trandolapril Cardiac Evaluation (TRACE) Study group. New Engl J Med 333(25): 1670–1676.

Levy D, Kenchaiah S, Larson MG, et al. (2002) Long-term trends in the incidence of and survival with heart failure. New Engl J Med 347(18): 1397–1402.

Møller JE, Brendorp B, Ottesen M, et al. (2003) Congestive heart failure with preserved left ventricular systolic function after acute myocardial infarction: clinical and prognostic implications. Eur J Heart Fail 5(6): 811–819.

Mehta R, Dabbous O, Granger C, et al. (2003) Comparision of outcomes of patients with acute coronary syndromes with and without atrial fibrillation. Am J Cardiol; 92: 1031–36.

NICE. (2006) Guidelines for ICD implantation. http://www.nice.org.uk/guidance/index.jsp?action=byID&o=11566, (accessed 13/02/08).

Nishimura R, Gersh BJ, Schaff HV, et al. (2000) The case for an aggressive surgical approach to papillary muscle rupture following myocardial infarction: 'From paradise lost to paradise regained'. Heart 83: 611–613.

Peter JV, Moran JL, Phillips-Hughes J, et al. (2006) Effect of non-invasive positive pressure ventilation (NIPPV) on mortality in patients with acute cardiogenic pulmonary oedema: a meta-analysis. Lancet 367: 1155–1163.

Pfeffer MA, McMurray JJ, Velazquez EJ, et al. (2003) Valsartan, captopril, or both in myocardial infarction complicated by heart failure, left ventricular dysfunction, or both. New Engl J Med 349(20): 1893–1906.

Pitt B, Remme W, Zannad F, et al. (2003) Eplerenone, a selective aldosterone blocker, in patients with left ventricular dysfunction after myocardial infarction. New Engl J Med 348: 1309–1321.

Roger VL, Weston SA, Redfield MM, et al. (2004) Trends in heart failure incidence and survival in a community-based population. J Am Med Assoc 292: 344–350.

Rutherford JD, Pfeffer MA, Moyé LA, et al. (1994) Effects of captopril on ischaemic events after myocardial infarction. Results of the Survival and Ventricular Enlargement trial. SAVE Investigators. Circulation 90(4): 1731–1738.

Chapter 8

Cardiac rehabilitation

Andrew A. McCleod

> **Key points**
> - Is a **vital** component of complete cardiac care.
> - Without Cardiac Rehabilitation the benefits of expensive modern therapy such as coronary stenting may not last.
> - Should involve the patient as an important manager of their own care.
> - Is multi-component, including drug therapy, specialized advice and support.
> - Includes exercise if at all possible because of proven benefits which may include molecular remodelling in diseased arteries.

8.1 Introduction

I didn't know what to do, Doc. I didn't know if I could walk upstairs. I didn't know if it was safe to make love to my wife. Then I came here, they put me on the treadmill, and I found I was OK.

(US post-heart–attack patient, Durham, North Carolina, 1981)

These were the words of a typical middle-aged male patient who had suffered a heart attack. When he had been discharged from his local hospital, his doctors had assured him he had made an excellent recovery from this event, and he could go back to normal. But as we can see from his remarks, his life had been dramatically changed and he was entering a new period of uncertainty where he did not know what was and what wasn't safe to do, and he did not really understand what had happened to him. Cardiac rehabilitation programmes were an early response in the USA to the growing awareness in the 1970s of treatment requirements of patients who had left hospital after a heart attack. In different formats they are now found in every country with a high prevalence of coronary artery disease (CAD). In this chapter I try to summarize what is known about cardiac rehabilitation, and future directions for research and improvement.

8.2 **A definition**

The following definition is that of the World Health Organization (WHO, 1993):

> *The rehabilitation of cardiac patients is the sum of activities required to influence favourably the underlying cause of the disease, as well as the best possible physical, mental, and social conditions, so that they may by their own efforts preserve, or resume when lost, as normal a place as possible in the community. Rehabilitation cannot be regarded as an isolated form of therapy, but must be integrated with the whole treatment of which it forms only one facet.*

8.3 **History**

The WHO definition of cardiac rehabilitation (CR) encompasses most of the goals of a good programme, but it was only arrived at following a process of evolution.

In the second half of the 20th century, the most widely recognized manifestation of coronary artery disease was the heart attack or myocardial infarction. The earlier term 'coronary thrombosis' was replaced by 'myocardial infarction' when flawed pathological studies suggested that the infarct-related artery was often not occluded by clot at post mortem. The phenomenon of late clot lysis was not understood, a factor which retarded the development of treatments such as thrombolysis and immediate coronary angioplasty. The development of coronary care units to watch for, and treat with immediate defibrillation, the complication of ventricular fibrillation (VF) focused attention on in-hospital management of this condition. Its aftermath, following recovery, was first modified by Samuel Levine and Bernard Lown, who pioneered the 'chair treatment of acute coronary thrombosis'. Getting the patient out of bed became the first step to a more enlightened approach to management.

In the 1940s and 1950s, it was realized that the frequency of this modern epidemic resulted in enormous economic loss, as experienced and successful workers were rarely returning to work. Work classification clinics in the USA successfully enabled the utilization of what was termed 'residual capacity' of the heart to achieve re-employment, or modification of work duties for many patients. This approach reversed what had been termed 'vocational death'.

In the 1960s and 1970s, research focused on the enhancement of reserve capacity and improved physical fitness. Studies of physical training in coronary artery disease patients demonstrated improvement in parameters related to coronary risk, for example clotting factors, blood pressure, and lipids. Other factors, such as weight loss or the prescription of recently proven beneficial drugs (beta-blockers), might have influenced the apparently beneficial results of trials conducted in CR patients.

This era culminated in two meta-analyses of CR studies, both published in the late 1980s, clearly showing that the overall effect of CR was a follow-up mortality reduction for post-myocardial infarction patients of around 20 per cent. A more recent review for the Cochrane collaboration suggests that exercise alone accounts for this benefit.

8.4 **Secondary disease prevention**

In the 21st century, we should not become overly messianic about the benefits of any one intervention for CAD patients. It is clear that secondary prevention of progressive or recurrent CAD is vital, and this includes the following drugs.

8.4.1 **Aspirin**

Aspirin is the oldest synthetic compound. Originally an analgesic, it is now important in therapy because it reduces risk of recurrent coronary thrombosis, via an effect of reversible inhibition of platelet cyclooxygenase.

8.4.2 **Clopidogrel**

Clopidogrel is a thienopyridine. These drugs inhibit platelet activation via the ADP receptor. Theoretical considerations suggested they should be less useful than inhibitors of the GPIIb/IIIa receptor, but oral studies with GPIIb/IIIa blockers have shown no benefit from these drugs, whereas trials with thienopyridines now show benefit in ST-elevated myocardial infarction (STEMI) and Non-ST elevated myocardial infarction (NSTEMI), and routinely following percutaneous coronary intervention (PCI). The optimum duration of treatment has still to be defined, particularly following implantation of drug-eluting intracoronary stents.

8.4.3 **Statins**

Statins were first conclusively proven to reduce coronary events and mortality in 1994 in Scandinavia (in the 4S trial). The predominant benefit is mediated by lowering of low-density lipoprotein (LDL) cholesterol due to inhibition of the liver enzyme, HMG CoA reductase.

8.4.4 **Other lipid-modifying drugs**

8.4.4.1 *Cholesterol absorption inhibitors*

A new class of drugs, the cholesterol absorption inhibitors (representative drug ezetimibe), offers substantial promise in combination with statins. The enterohepatic circulation of cholesterol appears to be a useful target for treatment. Large-scale trial data are awaited.

8.4.4.2 *Fibrates*

Fibrates were among the earliest of lipid-modifying drugs. The effects of fibrates appear to be modest in comparison with statins, and there is no indication for their routine use. Gemfibrozil appears effective in subjects with isolated low high-density lipoprotein-cholesterol (HDL-C).

8.4.4.3 *HDL-raising drugs*

Nicotinic acid was first investigated in the Coronary Drug Project in the 1960s. Side effects preclude its routine use, but an anti-prostaglandin inhibitor to reduce flushing and headache in combination is in trial in the UK (HPS2-THRIVE).

8.4.4.4 *Omega-3 fatty acids*

Incorporation into fat modifies the type of storage triglyceride, with consequent haemorrheological and other molecular effects. A single very large study in Italy (GISSI-Prevenzione) shows reduction in mortality post-myocardial infarction. Current advice is to simulate the effects by increased intake of oily fish, though this seems an unlikely aspiration for most patients.

8.4.4.5 *Plant stanols*

These sterol compounds reduce cholesterol absorption and lower LDL cholesterol. They are available in proprietary products. There are potential interactions with human sterol biosynthesis, though subjects with atherosclerotic disease would probably have a favourable risk: benefit ratio.

8.4.5 **Beta-blockers**

Beta-blockers were first used as anti-anginal and anti-hypertensive drugs, and extensive studies show reduction in mortality after myocardial infarction, particularly when there is left ventricular impairment or overt cardiac failure. Side effects are often over-emphasized in the press. In double-blind trials in Europe, UK doctors consistently withdrew more patients on beta-blockers than doctors from other European countries, indicating that UK doctors are more prejudiced against these drugs than doctors in other countries.

8.4.6 **ACE inhibitors**

These drugs show clear reduction in mortality for patients with left ventricular dysfunction or heart failure. Some studies suggest a reduction in atherosclerotic complications and progression to Type 2 diabetes in angiotensin converting enzyme (ACE) inhibitor-treated patients. In snormotensive, non-diabetic patients with normal left ventricular function there is little evidence to mandate routinely prescribing these drugs or the newer angiotensin receptor blockers.

8.4.7 **Diuretics**

Because oral diuretic drugs have been available for symptomatic relief of oedema for many years, they have not been subjected to double-blind scrutiny in trials. Nonetheless, in studies, patients on ACE inhibitors and diuretics for cardiac impairment who had the diuretic withdrawn showed deterioration in symptoms and left ventricular function.

8.4.8 **Aldosterone blockade**

Secondary hyperaldosteronism in heart failure patients probably limits the benefit of the ACE inhibitors and other vasodilators. Patients on long-term treatment with ACE inhibitors show a phenomenon of 'aldosterone escape', where previously low levels of aldosterone rise towards pre-treatment levels. This therefore probably underlies the remarkably positive benefits shown in the Randomized Aldactone Evaluation Study (RALES) trial, using spironolactone therapy in patients who had hospital admissions and were in NYHA Class III or IV heart failure (30 per cent mortality reduction). Spironolactone, a drug produced half a century ago, also has anti-androgenic activity, which produces significant side effects such as gynaecomastia in men. Eplerenone, a more recently available specific aldosterone inhibitor, is of proven benefit in patients who have heart failure after myocardial infarction (EPHESUS trial).

8.4.9 **Coumarin anticoagulants**

Studies with these drugs in coronary artery disease go back half a century with phenindione, and more recently with warfarin. Warfarin remains one of the few drugs whose dosage is determined routinely by its effect. There is little evidence for its routine use in post-myocardial infarction patients, though a good study in Norway showed benefit in 'high-risk' patients. A consensus would recommend its use in CAD patients with atrial fibrillation, demonstrated left ventricular aneurysm or mural thrombus, and possibly severe heart failure with immobility.

8.4.10 **Erythrocyte stimulation**

Anaemia is a feature of advanced heart failure. The coronary circulation is unique in its ability to extract oxygen maximally from haemoglobin. Coronary sinus blood has a lower oxygen saturation than venous blood from any other body tissue. A corollary of this is that unlike peripheral muscle, which adapts with exercise training (see section 8.6), increased oxygen delivery to the myocardium can only occur when red cell mass is increased. These treatments are beyond the scope of this review.

8.5 **Other components of cardiac rehabilitation**

The British Association for Cardiac Rehabilitation (BACR) has followed the lead of other national societies and published a set of standards and core components for cardiac rehabilitation (BACR 2007). Recommended staffing includes specialist nurses, physiotherapists, dietitians, pharmacists, and clinical psychologists. The role of each of these will be briefly examined in turn.

8.5.1 **Specialist nursing**

Specialist nursing staff will often have a background in cardiac nursing, which is an ideal preparation for working with patients in the months and years following presentation with cardiac disease. Their knowledge of all components of care is wide-ranging. In less well funded programmes their role will include all of the other skills given below.

8.5.2 **Physiotherapist or exercise specialist**

A degree of specialization in cardiac problems is essential. Postgraduate courses exist for training in this field.

8.5.3 **Dietitian**

Changing dietary pattern is one of the hardest things to achieve. Perhaps the common experience of not achieving weight loss in patients who clearly require it underpins the reluctance of funding authorities to invest in dietitians. Nonetheless, published data from Dean Ornish in California (the Lifestyle Heart Trial) show what can be achieved in an enclosed environment with dietary modification.

8.5.4 **Clinical psychologist**

The work of a clinical psychologist overlaps that of other personnel. A significant minority of cardiac patients suffer from overt depression, and depressed patients consistently do badly clinically. They fail to take lifestyle advice (dietary modification, exercise, and smoking cessation) and may not be compliant with medication. Very little investment in services for depressed patients exists in the UK. Patients often have misapprehensions about their condition which must be corrected. In addition, many patients are concerned about potential or real sexual difficulties following detection of CAD, and are reluctant to discuss these unless given a sympathetic opportunity to do so.

The role of a psychologist can be, and often is, assumed by medical and nursing staff. The process by which a staff member can act as a role model and resource for a patient is an important one, and overlaps with the psychological discipline of cognitive behavioural therapy. In this technique, the therapist seeks to facilitate the achievement of lifestyle change for the patient by a process of self-examination, understanding the nature of the disease, goal-setting, and learning techniques for achieving the goals set. Merely instructing the patient what he or she should do, the traditional way for a doctor to manage a case, is rarely successful. The thrust for improvement in the condition is a process of self-management. Those treating coronary artery disease patients have belatedly come to the realization which diabetologists have propounded for many years, namely that the most important person in the management of the condition is the patient. Self-help is therefore important, but can be underpinned by an experienced therapist, for example in the approach of the Heart Manual (1992), which is widely available in Scotland.

8.6 **Exercise**

No change in the last hundred years has been so dramatic as the reduction in exercise taken by Western populations, together with a remarkable availability of food. Indeed, it has been said that the problems of half of the world are due simply to want, and of the other half due to excess. Recent studies on the spiralling levels of obesity interestingly show that caloric excess compared with intake 50 years ago is less of an issue than the continued decline in caloric consumption by lack of exercise. What are the mechanisms by which exercise benefits cardiac patients?

Used in conjunction with a better approach to diet, exercise can lower body weight and therefore the risk of associated conditions such as hypertension, arthritis, hyperlipidaemia, and Type 2 diabetes. Remarkably, exercise *per se* appears to be highly effective in reducing the likelihood of Type 2 diabetes.

Aerobic exercise is defined as a level of exertion with steady-state increased oxygen uptake compared with resting uptake, which can be maintained for long periods of time. Clearly, sprinting and short- to middle-distance running are not steady-state exercise, whereas vigorous, sustained exercise results in increased lactate levels produced by the exercising muscle, which are tolerated for long periods of time because their clearance (ultimately by complete oxidation) becomes equal to their production. The training effect of regular sustained vigorous exercise results in some important changes that can benefit cardiac patients. The level of exercise habit at which these effects occur appears to be a minimum of three sessions per week lasting 30 minutes or more, and sustained at about 60 to 85 per cent of maximal aerobic capacity, which is measured as overall oxygen uptake.

8.6.1 **Central haemodynamics**

After exercise training, maximal oxygen uptake is enhanced by development within muscle cells at the organelle level (e.g. development of mitochondria) and at the cellular level (e.g. increased capillarization of muscle tissue). Improved oxygen delivery can thus be achieved at lower blood flows than previously. Muscle tissue can therefore be perfused at a lower heart rate and blood pressure to achieve the same level of external work. Heart rate and blood pressure (after-load) are two key determinants of myocardial oxygen demand. A trained patient can thus perform a level of external work that he or she could not achieve previously without cardiac limitation. Excellent studies show reduced myocardial ischaemia during everyday activity after exercise training. In patients with very impaired myocardial function, this peripheral training effect can enhance quality of life and independent functioning.

8.6.2 **Molecular effects**

In atherosclerotic arteries, a variety of adverse biochemical effects occur. Some of these are still incompletely understood but relate to reduced capacity to lyse thrombus, enhanced platelet activation, and reduced ability to prevent thrombus formation. Arteries also react paradoxically to vasodilator stimuli with acetylcholine, constricting instead of relaxing. Recent work in Germany has shown that exercise training can induce genes which return this response to normal, enhancing tissue perfusion and reducing ischaemia. Despite the dramatic change in the angiographic appearance of a coronary artery after intervention with dilatation and intracoronary stenting, the vessel wall remains abnormal, and therapeutic intervention is still necessary to reduce risk of restenosis and thrombosis. Exercise training may therefore add to the more obvious benefits of percutaneous treatment of CAD.

8.6.3 **Dose of exercise**

Some of the studies quoted above have used quite intense regimes of aerobic exercise. The Leipzig studies of molecular change within the vessel wall used daily intensive aerobic exercise on a bicycle ergometer. Countries such as Germany often employ an in-patient approach to cardiac rehabilitation, which favours an intensive multi-disciplinary approach. Recent audit of CR programmes in the UK suggests that, whether due to lack of trainers or facilities, the dose of exercise administered to patients is less than that studied in the randomized trials on which the evidence base rests. Some well-intentioned programmes in the UK therefore may be offering little other than psychological support, education, and an audit of secondary prevention therapy.

8.6.3.1 *How to determine the dose of exercise*

There is a remarkably consistent relationship between the myocardial oxygen requirement to pump blood to exercising muscles (certainly during large muscle-mass exercise), and the level of external work done. Heart rate in turn is generally linearly related to the level of myocardial oxygen uptake. Maximal heart rate varies from person to person (standard deviation about 10 beats per minute) but is closely allied to age, falling steadily from the age of about 20 years. Ideally, the measurement of the difference between resting and maximal heart rate should be measured during aerobic (e.g. treadmill or bicycle ergometer) exercise. The chosen steady-state target (e.g. 75 per cent) can then be chosen from a graph (the Karvonen method). This ratio remains reliable even when patients are taking heart-rate–modifying drugs such as beta-blockers, though of course the exercise assessment for determination of heart rate then needs to be performed on therapy. Gunnar Borg realized that the subjective level of exercise can be recognized by the subject and reliably related to the level of external work (the Borg Scale). With practice, exercising subjects can substitute a Borg Scale rating for a measured heart rate. Access to cheap and reliable heart-rate monitors, however, makes the Borg Scale less important than it previously was.

8.6.4 **Epidemiologic evidence**

A very large body of evidence underpins the observation that increased physical activity reduces CAD mortality. The more sophisticated studies clearly show that this is not confounded by a tendency for those with higher risk of CAD to take less exercise than those with inherent lower risk. In addition, longitudinal studies of those who have not exercised when younger, but who take up exercise later in life, show that a protective effect can be obtained later, compared with those who have continued to take less exercise.

In patients with CAD, there is overwhelming evidence of benefit. Exercise does not appear to be associated with increased risk for cardiac patients. Those who take the least exercise, but who suddenly undertake violent physical effort, can trigger cardiac events. In extreme circumstances this probably results from direct rupture of a fragile fibrous cap over an atheromatous plaque. Most studies of exercise in vulnerable patients, e.g. those with pre-existing cardiac failure, suggest that it can be undertaken safely. The overall effect of CR in improving mortality is probably multi-factorial, and results from exercise, appropriate indivualized therapy, and encouragement and support to make lifestyle changes such as improvement in diet, smoking cessation, and weight reduction.

8.7 **Conclusion**

This review does not address the complexities of exercise training in vulnerable patient groups. Special precautions may be necessary in heart failure patients, such as arrhythmia monitoring. Disabled and elderly patients need tailored approaches. Nonetheless, care of any patient with CAD must focus on the long-term element of the disease.

There are strong commercial imperatives that keep interventional and therapeutic devices and drugs in the public mind. What determines the long-term outcome for the patient, however, may be the elements of care that make up the much longer period of time after the brief encounter with secondary and tertiary care services in hospital.

Key references

Astrand P-O, Rodahl K, Dahl HA, Strømme SB. (2003) *Textbook of work physiology: physiological bases of exercise*, 4th edn. Human Kinetics, Champaign, USA.

Balady GJ, Williams MA, Ades PA, *et al.* (2007) Core components of cardiac rehabilitation/secondary prevention programmes: 2007 update. *Circulation* **115**: 2675–2682.

British Association for Cardiac Rehabilitation (BACR). (2007) *Standards and Core Components for Cardiac Rehabilitation*. http://www.bcs.com/documents/affiliates/bacr/BACR%20standards%202007.pdf (accessed 14/01/08).

Cardiac Rehabilitation. Scottish Intercollegiate Guidelines Network (SIGN). (2002) *Guideline No. 57*. http://www.sign.ac.uk/guidelines/fulltext/57/index.html (accessed 14/01/08).

Haskell WL, Lee I-M, Pate RR, *et al.* (2007) Physical activity and public health. Updated recommendation for adults from the American College of Sports Medicine and the American Heart Association. *Med Sci Sports Exerc;* **39**: 1423–34.

NHS Lothian. (1992) The Heart Manual. http://www.theheartmanual.com/ (accessed 14/01/08).

McLeod AA. (2002) Evidentiary basis for non-pharmacological intervention: effective management of lifestyle and associated risk factors. In: *Effective secondary prevention and cardiac rehabilitation* (eds Wood D, McLeod A, Davis M, Miles A), pp. 17–37. UK Key Advances in Clinical Practice Series. Aesculapius Medical Press, London.

Chapter 9

Follow-up: the specialist's perspective

Peter Henriksen, Nick Boon

Key points

- There is no need for continuous follow-up of acute coronary syndrome patients.
- At least one follow-up appointment is helpful to ensure that:
  - any ongoing symptoms are addressed.
  - plans are in place to manage any residual disease not treated at the time of the index event.
  - optimum anti-thrombotic therapy is prescribed.
  - all cardiovascular risk factors are addressed as far as possible.
- The clinic letter should list all current medications and describe clearly any proposed changes, together with any plans for further investigation or treatment.
- On discharge from the clinic, the patient should be advised on what to do in the event of recurrent or worsening symptoms.

9.1 The rationale of the follow-up clinic

9.1.1 Planned review

The biology of atherosclerosis and the unpredictable nature of its complications make regular clinic review in the hospital outpatient department illogical. However, it is important to formally evaluate a patient's progress following an admission for treatment of an acute coronary syndrome in order to address any ongoing symptoms, determine if therapy for any residual disease manifesting as ischaemia or left ventricular dysfunction is required, optimize drug therapy and risk factor control, and ensure that appropriate rehabilitation is underway (Figure 9.1). Clinical audit and research can also be continued at the review clinic. Although follow-up usually takes place in a hospital outpatient clinic, many patients could be managed in specialist primary care clinics. Only one clinic visit may be necessary for patients who have had an uncomplicated admission. Many therapies are evidence-based and directed by guidelines and protocols which should be accessible in the clinic, preferably on-line, together with relevant clinical details and blood results.

Patients who have presented with an acute coronary syndrome will have a life-long elevated risk of recurrent events and should be targeted for aggressive risk factor control. Setting the timing of outpatient review at three to four months following discharge allows assessment for recurrent symptoms related to the development of restenosis in patients who have had percutaneous intervention and allows the clinician to assess the impact of rehabilitation programmes that will be nearing completion.

9.1.2 **Unplanned review**

The development of new or worsening symptoms of myocardial ischaemia always requires prompt clinical assessment. The patient should receive education before discharge (both following hospital admission and from clinic) on what action to take in the event of recurrent symptoms. Intense chest discomfort lasting more than 10 to 15 minutes despite glyceryl trinitrate (GTN) spray warrants an

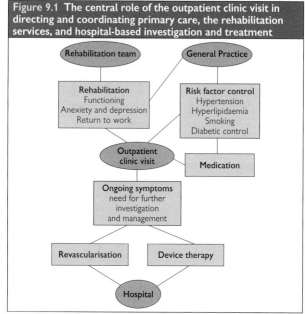

Figure 9.1 The central role of the outpatient clinic visit in directing and coordinating primary care, the rehabilitation services, and hospital-based investigation and treatment

emergency call for an ambulance. A deterioration in chest pain symptoms without prolonged episodes at rest can be further assessed by the general practitioner. Depending on clinical presentation the patient may require immediate assessment in hospital on the same day or prompt review in an emergency clinic within two to three days. Adjustment of medication may be all that is necessary for patients with very mild symptoms prior to routine review in the cardiology clinic.

9.2 Management of ongoing symptoms and residual disease

A detailed symptom history should be taken together with a directed physical examination looking for evidence of myocardial ischaemia and complications such as congestive cardiac failure and arrhythmias.

9.2.1 Residual coronary disease

Patients with ongoing angina symptoms following an acute coronary syndrome episode are at high risk of myocardial infarction (MI) and should be considered for angiography with a view to revascularization.

Information on residual coronary disease will be available if the patient has had coronary angiography during their admission. If the patient is stable and has severe residual disease that is amenable to revascularization, an elective procedure (either percutaneous or surgical) can be arranged; this is often undertaken approximately 6 weeks after the index event to allow sufficient time for the culprit lesion and any infarcted myocardium to heal. For asymptomatic patients with residual coronary disease, a conservative approach may be justified, particularly if the patient has returned to full activities. Stress testing with exercise ECG or perfusion imaging is helpful where there is doubt about the impact of residual disease. Evidence of asymptomatic ischaemia on stress testing merits consideration for further revascularization, particularly if the area of ischaemia is sub-stantial or the vessel involved has prognostic significance (e.g. proximal segment of left anterior descending vessel).

Patients who receive thrombolysis for ST-elevation myocardial infarction (STEMI) may not have had coronary angiography during their index admission and should undergo some form of stress testing at follow-up. Patients admitted with unstable angina and identified as being at low risk on the basis of clinical markers may also not have undergone coronary angiography and should undergo stress testing if this was not performed prior to discharge from the ward.

9.2.2 Left ventricular impairment

Symptoms of congestive cardiac failure may not be identified until the patient increases activity following discharge. Patients with symp-tomatic left ventricular dysfunction are in an adverse prognostic group and merit particularly close monitoring. Echocardiography provides useful information on regional wall motion abnormalities and valvular dysfunction, including ischaemic mitral regurgitation, which may be significant despite an absence of clinical signs. Management of post-infarct heart failure is discussed fully in Chapter 7.

The follow-up clinic provides an opportunity to select patients for automatic implantable cardioverter-defibrillator (AICD) implantation. National Institute for Health and Clinical Excellence (NICE) guidance on AICD implantation for primary prevention against sudden arrhythmic death was issued in 2006. This indicates that all patients with a severely depressed ejection fraction (less than 30 per cent) and a QRS duration on the ECG of greater than 120 milliseconds and who have survived more than 4 weeks from a myocardial infarct with no worse than NYHA grade III heart failure symptoms should be considered for an AICD.

9.3 **Review of medications and risk factor control**

The patient's medication list should be reviewed in the follow-up clinic. There may be changes from the prescription issued on the ward at the time of discharge. The reason for a change in prescription should be identified (e.g. the development of side effects, a brand preference on the part of the primary care prescriber or simply the patient being unaware that the medication was to continue). It is often helpful to ask the patient, or their carer, to write down a list of their current medication on the day of the clinic visit or, if uncertain, to bring all their medications to clinic. The plans for continued anti-thrombotic treatment and risk factor control are of primary importance and must be addressed during the consultation.

9.3.1 **Anti-thrombotic treatment**

Dual anti-platelet therapy with aspirin and clopidogrel is indicated in all patients presenting with acute coronary syndromes. In the CURE trial, clopidogrel (75 mg od) was administered in addition to aspirin (75 mg od) for between 3 and 12 months. Clinical benefits were predominantly seen in the first 3 months of therapy and coronary intervention was not performed routinely in high-risk patients. This may have lead to overestimation of clopidogrel's effect in contemporary practice where intervention is routine. Current Scottish Intercollegiate Guideline Network (SIGN) guidelines advocate dual anti-platelet therapy for three months following a non-ST–elevation myocardial infarction. A one-month course of clopidogrel is recommended for patients who have received thrombolysis for ST-elevation myocardial infarction. For patients who have had coronary stenting in the context of an acute coronary syndrome, a three-month course of dual anti-platelet therapy is indicated for bare metal stents and 12 months for drug-eluting stents. Premature interruption of anti-platelet therapy, particularly within the first month, is a strong risk factor for acute stent thrombosis, which carries a mortality of 40 per cent. The importance of complying with therapy must therefore be emphasized to the patient.

Patients on long-term anti-coagulation therapy who have had an acute coronary syndrome must have anti-thrombotic therapy tailored according to the need for anti-coagulation, balanced against the increased risk of haemorrhage associated with aspirin and/or clopidogrel in combination with warfarin. Aspirin and warfarin combined reduce the incidence of myocardial infarction and ischaemic stroke compared with aspirin alone but this comes with an increased risk of major haemorrhage and no overall effect on mortality. Warfarin combined with aspirin is inferior to dual anti-platelet therapy in the prevention of acute stent thrombosis. Patient preference and whether therapy can be delivered safely should both be taken into account. For patients with atrial fibrillation it may be possible to stop warfarin for the duration of dual anti-platelet therapy. Patients remaining on warfarin who have had coronary stenting will generally be continued on one anti-platelet agent.

9.3.2 Medication for risk factor control

Patients admitted with acute coronary syndromes should be started on a statin prior to hospital discharge. Monitoring of the response to lipid-lowering therapy should be performed three months after any treatment change and is usually conducted by general practice. The 2005 Joint British Societies' guidelines recommend a target total cholesterol of less than 4 mmol/L and low-density lipoprotein (LDL) cholesterol of less than 2 mmol/L.

Hypertension should be treated aggressively, with a target of 130/80 mmHg. Blood pressure response to changes in therapy should be monitored for two to four weeks by general practice before introducing further changes in medication. Beta-blockers have protective effects in post-MI patients, particularly in the context of left ventricular failure. They are also the treatment of choice in patients with residual angina and hypertension.

Left ventricular impairment and diabetes mellitus are clear indications for ACE inhibitor treatment. The Heart Outcomes Prevention Evaluation (HOPE) and European trial On Reduction Of cardiac events with Perindopril in stable coronary Artery disease (EUROPA) trials suggested a benefit of long-term ACE inhibitor therapy in patients with stable coronary disease and it is reasonable to extrapolate these results to higher-risk patients with acute coronary syndromes.

Good glycaemic control reduces microvascular complications in both Type 1 and Type 2 diabetes. There is less evidence that glycaemic control reduces recurrent myocardial infarction in acute coronary syndrome patients. Indeed, the Diabetes Mellitus Insulin-Glucose Infusion in Acute Myocardial Infarction (DIGAMI) 2 trial failed to demonstrate a reduction in mortality or non-fatal cardiovascular events following three months of insulin therapy in patients presenting with acute myocardial infarction who had on admission a glucose level greater than 11.1 mmol/L. There is, however, good evidence that metformin is associated with reduced cardiovascular events and mortality compared with insulin or sulphonylureas; it should therefore be first-line treatment in patients with Type 2 diabetes and a body mass index greater than 25.

9.3.3 **Smoking cessation**

It is the responsibility of all health-care professionals to provide opportunistic advice and reiterate the health hazards associated with smoking. Patients with acute coronary syndromes are a particularly high-risk group and their prognosis will improve if they quit. If the patient is motivated to stop they should be supported with behavioural therapy and pharmacotherapy. Reasons for lack of motivation should be explored and the link between ongoing smoking and further coronary events should be emphasized. Nicotine replacement therapy may be commenced safely in most patients with acute coronary syndromes; although caution is advised in patients with unstable coronary disease, it is preferable to continued smoking. Bupropion and varenicline are additional agents that offer higher smoking cessation rates in conjunction with smoking cessation counselling. The latter should be available at a specialized clinic within the hospital or primary care.

9.4 **Rehabilitation**

Rehabilitation care including patient education, lifestyle modification, psychological support, and exercise training reduces mortality and is appreciated by patients. This subject is covered in detail in Chapter 8. The British Heart Foundation (BHF) publishes a series of patient information leaflets which may be particularly useful to reinforce lifestyle advice (Figure 9.2). These may be used to reinforce important messages about diet, physical activity, and cholesterol or to provide further background information on treatments such as angioplasty, bypass surgery, and defibrillator implantation. The follow-up clinic provides an opportunity to assess progress and identify problems. Structured exercise classes generally start four weeks after an acute coronary syndrome and have an important confidence-building role. Formal exercise testing may be performed in the hospital clinic prior to entering the rehabilitation programme to determine if patients who have had complicated admissions with heart failure or ventricular arrhythmias are suitable for exercise therapy.

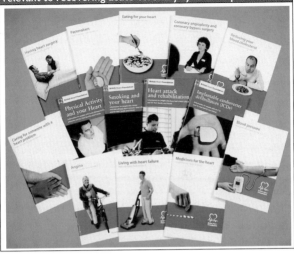

Figure 9.2 The BHF publishes booklets on a range of topics relevant to recovering acute coronary syndrome patients

Patients with persistent psychological symptoms, including depression and anxiety, may need referral for additional support. Reasons for not returning to work should be identified and addressed where possible. For patients with physically demanding work, liaison with an occupational health physician may be necessary. In the UK, to maintain a DVLA Group 2 driving licence for heavy goods or passenger vehicles, patients are currently required to complete nine minutes of the Bruce treadmill protocol safely, having stopped anti-anginal therapy such as beta-blockers 48 hours previously.

9.5 **The follow-up clinic letter**

Placing follow-up plans and recommendations on-line so that all members of the health-care team can access them allows expeditious and reliable communication of information. Moreover, this can be linked to databases and allows reference to guidelines and possible drug interactions, facilitates automatic electronic prompts and alerts, and is a powerful tool for audit and research. Nevertheless, most communication is still conducted by letter.

The clinic letter provides a summary of the consultation and should be concise; it will be read by the general practitioner and members of the rehabilitation team but also provides a point of reference for future outpatient appointments and hospital admissions.

The letter should list all important diagnoses and details of any revascularization procedure, including the vessels that have been treated and the type of stent (drug-eluting or bare metal) or graft (venous or arterial) that has been used. A complete list of medication and doses must be provided, with a brief summary of recommended changes to medication and plans for further investigation, revascularization or follow-up.

Key references

Boyle R. (2000) Cardiac rehabilitation. In: *Coronary heart disease: national service framework for coronary heart disease. Modern standards and service models.* http://www.dh.gov.uk/prod_consum_dh/groups/dh_dig_italassets/@dh/@en/documents/digitalasset/dh_4057524.pdf (accessed 13/01/08).

Cross X, Gaunt M. (2002) Dictating an outpatient letter. *Br Med J* **324**: S92.

Drivers' Medical Group, DVLA. (2007) *At a glance guide to the current medical standards for fitness to drive.* http://www.dvla.gov.uk/media/pdf/medical/aagv1.pdf (accessed 22/10/07).

Erne P, Schoenenberger AW, Burckhardt D, et al. (2007) Effects of percutaneous coronary interventions in silent ischaemia after myocardial infarction. The SWISSI II randomized control trial. *J Am Med Assoc* **297**: 1985–1991.

Joint British Societies 2. (2005) Joint British Societies' guidelines on prevention of cardiovascular disease in clinical practice. *Heart* **91**(suppl V): v29–v39.

Scottish Intercollegiate Guidelines Network 93. (2007) *Acute coronary syndromes.* http://www.sign.ac.uk/pdf/sign93.pdf (accessed 22/10/07).

Chapter 10

Follow-up: the general practitioner's perspective

Michael G. Kirby

Key points

- Follow-up of acute coronary syndrome patients is a key role for primary care.
- Funding is in place through the Quality and Outcomes Framework (QOF).
- Nurse-led clinics have been shown to be very effective.
- Prevention of further events will be of great importance to commissioning groups.
- Clear and comprehensive discharge information is essential, together with good communication lines between primary and secondary care.
- The National Institute for Health and Clinical Excellence (NICE) guidelines provide an excellent resource.

10.1 Introduction

Primary care has a key role to play in the follow-up of patients with cardiovascular disease. Cardiovascular disease is the major cause of premature death in most European and North American populations. In the UK the annual incidence is around 300,000, leading to 140,000 deaths. Stable angina is the most common symptom of cardiovascular disease, with around 20,000 new cases each year in the UK. Estimates for prevalence range from 1 million to nearly 2 million patients in the UK.

In the UK about 838,000 men and 394,000 women have had a myocardial infarction (MI) at some point in their lives, a total of 1.2 million people. Although death rates from coronary heart disease (CHD) have been falling since the early 1970s when compared internationally, the UK death rate from CHD remains high, with more than 103,000 deaths per year. These death rates vary with age, gender, socioeconomic status, ethnicity, and geographic location (NICE 2007). Primary care will have an intimate knowledge of many of these variables and this provides commissioning groups with an opportunity to examine preventative strategies.

The effective management of cardiovascular disease in primary care is essential and will be of great interest to commissioning groups. The main aim will be to prevent acute events, deterioration in symptoms, and admission to hospital, which is expensive.

10.2 **Hospital discharge**

The hospital discharge summary is a key document and will set the scene for continuing care once the patient gets home following a cardiovascular event. Clear, concise information is critical for the seamless transfer from secondary to primary care. Unfortunately there are serious problems with the validity of clinical information, particularly in interim discharge documents, which are usually hand-written and prepared by a junior doctor. Incomplete information poses problems for the receiving clinician and also for the National Health Service (NHS) central data returns. This clearly can affect resource management, performance indicators, and other secondary uses of health information (Williams & Mann 2002).

The final discharge summary is usually dictated and posted as a typed letter, although structured computer-generated discharge summaries are becoming more common and are probably less likely to be incomplete. Patients should be aware that personal information about them will be shared within the health-care teams and given the opportunity to object if they wish to do so. The patient should be given a copy of the clinical communication, unless it is clinically inappropriate to do so. Most patients like having information and find it helpful (Sandler et al. 1989).

Patient care may be affected if complete discharge information is not available when the patient is next seen. Historically this has been an area of great concern (Harding 1987, Lockwood & Callum 1970, Mageean 1986). One randomized controlled trial found that the use of a computer-database–generated summary resulted in more discharge documents being produced within 4 weeks of discharge (Val Walraven et al. 1999). A smaller before-and-after study found that using an electronic system reduced the delay from 2.4 days to less than 1 hour (Branger et al. 1992). The transfer of discharge communication should contain information under the headings shown in Box 10.1, as recommended in SIGN 3.

Any drug reactions or other problems that developed during the hospital stay should be noted under current diagnoses, together with existing diagnosis on admission. Progress in hospital and any other clinically important information should be noted under the case review.

There should also be a management plan that should include specific instructions for the receiving doctor, any services provided, and follow-up requirements. Incorrect or irrelevant diagnoses are a common source of error and can lead to incorrect data being transcribed onto the primary care database (Adhiyaman et al. 2000).

> **Box 10.1 Discharge information**
>
> - Hospital
> - Patient ID (national ID, local ID, forename, surname, address, postcode, date of birth)
> - Preferred general practitioner (GP) ID
> - Consultant ID
> - Validating clinician
> - Patient's registered GP details
> - Admission details (administrative)
> - Discharge details (administrative)
> - Review of case
> - Current diagnosis
> - Allergies
> - Procedures and investigations
> - Medications and dietary requirements
> - Functional state
> - Systems review
> - Examination findings
> - Results of investigations
> - Problem list
> - Management plan
> - Intended outcomes
> - Information given to patient

10.3 **Primary care**

Chronic disease management accounts for up to 80 per cent of the daily work in primary care and there are many opportunities to help patients learn to live with their chronic illness (Department of Health 2000). Quality of life deteriorates significantly after a cardiovascular event, but this deterioration can be ameliorated with good care, and we should be aiming to attain the best possible quality of life (Colin-Thone & Belfield 2004).

10.3.1 **Management issues**

The management of patients with cardiovascular disease is complex and requires a multi-disciplinary approach. The practice team will include reception staff, who will check on accurate registration details and perform searches and audit, health-care assistants, who will perform some of the routine monitoring tasks, practice nurses, who will adopt protocols dealing with highly complex care and management pathways, and primary care physicians, who will be dealing with diagnosis, follow-up, and day-to-day care of the patients.

10.4 **National initiatives**

Cardiovascular disease has been a priority area for primary care organizations (PCOs) for the last 10 years and major improvements in care have already been achieved following publication of the National Service Framework (NSF) for CHD (Department of Health 2000). The NSF for coronary heart disease was published in March 2000 and details 12 standards for improved prevention, diagnosis, treatment, and rehabilitation and goals to secure fair access to high-quality services.

Campbell and co-workers (2005) demonstrated a considerable improvement in the management of these patients between the years 1998 and 2000, predating the NSF, and continued improvements have come with the new General Medical Services (GMS) contract and the Quality and Outcomes Framework (QOF). The GMS2 contract for GPs came into effect in April 2004 and evolved in partnership between the NHS confederation and the General Practitioner's Committee (GPC) of the British Medical Association (BMA).

The Quality and Outcomes Framework of the GMS contract promoted high-quality, cost-effective care. These targets aimed to provide incentives to review approaches to treatment and manage medicines cost-effectively. The importance of QOF is that it provided, for the first time, adequate funding to provide a more comprehensive care package for patients with the nominated disease. This led to new contracts for nurses, who have been the main providers of high-quality disease management clinics.

Points are provided for achieving goals. The payment per point currently stands at £124.60. Practices can earn a maximum of 1000 points. Management of diabetes attracts 93 points, hypertension 83 points, atrial fibrillation 30 points, smoking 68 points, stroke and transient ischaemic attack (TIA) 24 points, kidney disease 27 points, CHD 89 points, and heart failure 20 points. Clearly peripheral vascular disease is a major omission.

There has been slow and continuous improvement in the management of patients with cardiovascular disease since 1998, long before payment for QOF came into force. These improvements have contributed to a significant 40 per cent reduction in deaths from circulatory disease over this time.

The quality of data in the disease registers is of critical importance and data need to be kept up to date. It is paramount that only appropriate patients are included, that all are correctly coded, and that practices can check their register against the average prevalence rates. The prevalences for April 2006–07 were as shown in Table 10.1 (Quality Management and Analysis System (QMAS) 2007). The sum of registers is for all practices. The unadjusted prevalence equals the sum of registers for all practices divided by the sum of list sizes for all practices, expressed as a percentage.

Table 10.1 QMAS Disease and prevalence rates

Clinical area	Sum of register	Unadjusted prevalence
CHD	1,898,565	3.5%
Heart failure	419,856	0.8%
Stroke and TIA	863,873	1.6%
Hypertension	6,705,899	12.5%
Diabetes mellitus	1,961,976	3.7%
Chronic kidney disease	1,279,246	2.4%
Atrial fibrillation	692,054	1.3%

The whole practice team needs to be up-to-date with the information technology, which needs to include hospital data capture on a daily basis. There are many patients who fall across several different indicator groups. Many practices are moving towards combined clinics because the protocols overlap for patients with hypertension, diabetes, CHD, and kidney disease. Smoking is an important indicator. There are allowable exceptions from these registers, which include patients who refuse to attend three times, where it is not clinically appropriate, patients who have expressed informed dissent, patients who cannot tolerate the medication, and patients who are taking the maximum tolerated dose of medication. New patients can also be excluded from the register, but must have relevant measurements such as blood pressure reading within 3 months and meet clinical standards within 9 months.

The overall exception reporting rates for England in 2006/07 were low (5.5 per cent), with only 5 per cent of practices having overall exception rates higher than 10 per cent. The average exception rate for CHD was 7.38 per cent, for diabetes 6 per cent, for hypertension 2.46 per cent, for ventricular dysfunction 8.61 per cent, and for stroke 7.53 per cent. Although there has been much controversy regarding the cost of QOF, which in 2005/06 was £1.1 billion, the GPC estimates that, looking at hypertension alone, intervention saves 8,700 patients from serious ill-health over a 5-year period.

10.4.1 Nurse led clinics

In my own practice a nurse-led clinic was introduced in 2002 and this required considerable planning, involving GPs, nurses, health visitors, the phlebotomy manager, the practice manager, and reception staff. At the time the practice had 5 per cent of the practice population on the CHD register due to a large number of elderly patients registered at that time. This required more than 450 patients to be seen in the first year and 675 attended, with a mean age of 74 years. A subsequent audit showed significantly improved assessment, significantly increased prescribing, and improved targets.

The Assessment of Implementation Strategies (ASSIST) trial, published in the *British Medical Journal* in June 2001, was a randomized controlled trial that included 21 general practices in Warwickshire and 1,900 patients randomized to nurse clinic, GP clinic, or audit and feedback. The trial concluded that nurse clinics were as effective as GP clinics and probably more so. Nurse clinics certainly improved assessment compared to the control, but the clinics did not significantly change the targets achieved. However, subsequently (Murchie *et al.* 2003) in the *British Medical Journal* on 11 January 2003, a randomized controlled trial of the effectiveness of nurse-led clinics, with a 4.7 year follow-up. This showed at one year that nurse clinics improved lifestyle, aspirin use, and blood pressure and lipid management and that at 4.7 years, the nurse clinics reduced total deaths and coronary events significantly, with an odds ratio of 0.76.

10.4.2 **Secondary prevention**

Secondary prevention is clearly a priority. Lifestyle interventions need to be recommended for all and influenza vaccinations are important. Cardiac rehabilitation after a myocardial infarction can reduce the risk of further episodes. Such programmes include advice and help on exercise, diet, stress, and other aspects of getting back into full health following a heart attack. Many patients find the opportunity to talk to other patients who have suffered a similar event very helpful (Chambers *et al.* 2001).

The NICE post-MI guideline updates relevant sections of the NSF on coronary heart disease (NICE 2007). Recommendations within this updated guideline incorporate practical advice around lifestyle interventions and cardiac rehabilitation but extend beyond the boundaries of many traditional guidelines. The guideline focuses on patient-centred care, stating that treatment and care should take into account patients' individual needs and preferences. Good communication, supported by evidence-based information, is essential to allow patients to reach informed decisions about their care. Carers and relatives should have the opportunity to be involved in discussions unless the patient thinks it inappropriate. The key priorities for implementation are well suited to being incorporated into the structure of the protocols being currently used in primary care.

Many patients become both anxious and depressed after a myocardial infarction and it is important to involve partners and carers in the rehabilitation process. NICE Clinical Guidelines 22 and 23 are helpful with regard to patients with clinical anxiety or depression.

10.4.3 **Sexual activity**

Sexual activity often goes undiscussed, due to embarrassment on the part of both the patient and the health-care professional. However, more than 60 per cent of male patients will suffer from erectile dysfunction following MI (Hodges *et al.* 2007). It is therefore important to discuss sexual activity within the context of rehabilitation and aftercare, since patients can be reassured that after recovery, sexual activity presents no greater risk of triggering a subsequent MI than if they had never had an MI. Patients who have made an uncomplicated recovery can resume sexual activity when they feel comfortable to, usually after about 4 weeks. The use of a phosphodiesterase type 5 (PDE5) inhibitor is very useful in those patients who are stable. PDE5 inhibitors should be avoided in patients treated with nitrates and/or nicorandil because of the risk of hypotension.

The Joint British Societies (JBS2 2005) guidelines (Table 10.2) provide advice on optimal treatment standards, which should be achieved wherever possible.

10.4.4 Team work

The strength of primary care is teamwork, which increases the chances of successfully managing patients with cardiovascular disease, and carers and relatives are important members of the team. The prevention of recurrent events and recurrent admissions are related to the factors shown in Box 10.2.

10.5 Audit and review

Regular clinical audits will identify patients who have not been reviewed in the last 12 months and these patients can be invited to a review appointment by one of the nurses. Ideally blood tests should be performed before the appointment so results are available at the time to aid decision-making. Home visits may be appropriate for those patients who are unable to attend the practice. A personal phone call can sometimes make the difference between attendance and non-attendance.

Table 10.2 Audit and optimal treatment standards for CVD prevention in people with established atherosclerotic disease (JBS2)

Variable	Target	Standard
Blood pressure	<150/90 mmHg	Audit standard
	<140/85 mmHg	Optimal treatment standard
	<145/80 mmHg	Audit standard for diabetes
	<130/80 mmHg	Optimal treatment standard in diabetes mellitus and high CVD risk
Lipids	TC <5.0 mmol/L	Audit standard
	TC <4.0 mmol/L	Optimal treatment standard
	LDL-C <3.0 mmol/L	Audit standard
	LDL-C <2.0 mmol/L	Optimal treatment standard
Glucose	HbA1c <6.5%	

TC = total cholesterol; LDL-C = calculated LDL cholesterol

> **Box 10.2 Prevention factors**
> * Poor control of risk factors
> * Non-concordance with medication and lifestyle measures
> * Intercurrent infection
> * Failed social support
> * Psychosocial problems
> * Failure of follow-up

Ongoing training is essential for all team members to ensure accurate data entry, maintenance of disease registers, risk stratification, identification of key responsibilities, and ongoing medical education.

Communication between primary and secondary care is essential because effective treatment starts in hospital. Commissioning groups should ensure through contracts that joined-up thinking with regard to NICE guidance and regular audits will facilitate this process.

Key references

Adhiyaman V, Oke A, White AD. (2000) Diagnoses in discharge communications: how are they reliable? *Int J Clin Pract* **54**: 457–458.

Branger PJ, Van der Wouden JC, Schudel BR et al. (1992) Electronic communication between providers of primary and secondary care. *Br Med J* **305**: 1068–1070.

Campbell SM, O'Roland M, et al. (2005) Improvements in quality of clinical care in English general practice 1998–2003. *Br Med J* **331**: 1121–1123.

Chambers R, Wakeley G, Iqbal Z. (2001) *Cardiovascular matters in primary care*. Radcliffe Medical Press, Oxford.

Colin-Thone D, Belfield G. (2004) *Improving chronic disease management*. Department of Health, London.

Department of Health. (1999) *Saving lives: our healthier nation*. Executive summary. Department of Health, London.

Department of Health. (2000) *National Service Framework for coronary heart disease*. Department of Health, London.

Harding J. (1987) Study of discharge communications from hospital doctors to an inner London general practice. *J R Coll Gen Pract* **37**: 494–495.

Hodges LD, Kirby M, Solanki J, et al. (2007) The temporal relationship between erectile dysfunction and cardiovascular disease. *Int J Clin Pract* **61**(12): 2019–25.

Joint British Societies 2 (JBS2). (2005) Joint British Societies' guidelines on prevention of cardiovascular disease in clinical practice. *Heart* **91**(suppl. V):V1–V52.

Lockwood E, McCallum FM. (1970) Patients discharged from hospital: an aspect of communication in the Health Service. *Health Bull (Edinb)* **28**: 75–80.

Mageean RJ. (1986) Study of 'discharge communications' from hospital. *Br Med J (Clin Res Ed)* **293**: 1283–1284.

National Institute for Health and Clinical Excellence (NICE). (2007) *Clinical Guideline 48. MI: secondary prevention. Secondary prevention in primary and secondary care for patients following a myocardial infarction*. NICE, London.

QMAS. (2007) *QMAS Database 2006/07*. Information Centre for Health and Social Care, Prescribing Support Unit, London. www.ic.nhs.uk (accessed 12/01/08).

Sandler DA, Heaton C, Garner ST, Mitchell JR. (1989) Patients' and general practitioners' satisfaction with information given on discharge from hospital: audit of a new information card. *Br Med J* **299**: 1511–1513.

Van Walraven C, Laupacis A, Seth R, Wells G. (1999) Dictated versus database-generated discharge summaries: a randomised clinical trial. *CMAJ* **160**: 319–326.

Williams JG, Mann RY. (2002) Hospital episode statistics: time for clinicians to get involved. *Clin Med* **2**: 34–37.

Index